The Detox Diet

A How-to & When-to
Guide for Cleansing the Body

by

Elson M. Haas, MD

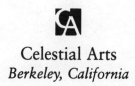

Celestial Arts
Berkeley, California

I would like to thank my publisher, David Hinds, and my editors, Veronica Randall and Christa Laib of Celestial Arts. Thank you also to Bethany ArgIsle and Nancy Faass for your helpful and insightful contributions. Also, I am thankful to Dr. Franz Morrell and Dr. Alexander Wood for the nutritional concepts that generated *The Detox Diet*.

Note: *Ending your addictions is a serious undertaking. Going "cold turkey" from sedatives, stimulants, narcotics, and alcohol can have very serious consequences, including seizures. There are many excellent doctors and facilities, including hospital detox centers, available to help us deal with drug and alcohol problems. This book is intended as a supplement, not a substitute, to the interventions of an experienced, professional healthcare practitioner.*

Celestial Arts Publishing
P.O. Box 7123
Berkeley, California 94707

Cover: Toni Tajima
Text: Shelley Firth

Library of Congress Catalog Card Number: 96 - 84976

Printed in the United States

First Printing, 1996
    3 4 / 99 98 97

Table of Contents

◆

Renewal

◆

So many problems in Western society come from the excessive use of food and drugs. Abuses and addictions touch almost every person's life. I realize that the development of these habits is multi-faceted and as much a part of our social and cultural upbringing as they are our responses to dealing with a stressful family, school, work, and society at large.

I don't want you to feel bad, weak, or inferior if any of these potentially destructive habits applies to you. I know the struggle between light and dark—between picking up that cup of coffee or glass of wine or that pack of cigarettes and the desire to stop or to never have started. I also know that it is an incredible challenge to change anything—particularly to clear any habit/abuse/addiction that we have had years to get used to and rely upon. I have seen that it can be done with greater attentiveness to ourselves, with a gathering of our willpower, and with the support of our loved ones. And I have also seen that it is very difficult without a willingness to deal openly with emotions and other adversaries that may block our way toward healing.

I do want to inspire and motivate you to change. The first principle for improving your health is to eliminate destructive habits. Even if you cannot fathom at this time doing without your substances completely, at least consider an "abuse break." Try a day or week without caffeine, alcohol, or sugar, replacing them with a new habit—drinking water, walking, or swimming, for example.

All addictions are ultimately self-destructive (some can hurt others as well, such as alcohol and smoking). When you change that dynamic to self care—through both your internal healing process as well as with the lifestyle and nutritional guidelines I describe in this book—you will begin to serve your body and life toward its highest potential. As you develop more nurturing and supportive habits—eating good food, exercising regularly, learning to cope with stress, and developing motivating attitudes—I can promise you will experience greater vitality, more positive relationships, and overall improved health.

Good luck on your journey.

Before You Begin

◆

As a physician, I am fascinated by the complexity, subtlety, and diversity of individual health habits—the combinations of the various substances we imbibe and ingest. The spectrum of these substances includes the components of our diet (foods, drinks, chemicals), supplements (nutrients, herbs, homeopathics), drugs (prescription, over-the-counter, and recreational), and pollutants (herbicides, pesticides, hydrocarbons, and petrochemicals).

How do we develop our preferences? When do our preferences become needs? Why do our needs become addictions? Why do some of us become addicted while others can stop on their own? Our personality, upbringing, and our environment influence our personal choice of substances. In exploring these concerns about abuse and the way it affects our health, I have developed a specific orientation and program for initial healing and detoxification. This process has evolved over my twenty-five years as a naturally-based general health practitioner.

My overall understanding of symptoms and disease integrates both Western linear thinking and naturopathic approaches to health and illness. Problems with the body and mind often arise from either **deficiency** (when we are not acquiring sufficient nutrients to meet our bodily needs) and/or **congestion** (when our intake is excessive). Congestion involves both reduced eliminative function and an overconsumption of food or substances, such as caffeine, alcohol, nicotine, refined sugar, and chemicals.

People who are deficient may experience problems such as fatigue, coldness, hair loss, or dry skin. They need to be nourished with wholesome foods that aid healing. However, congestive problems are more common in Western, industrialized countries. Many of our acute and chronic diseases result from clogged tissues, suffocated cells, and subsequent loss of vital energy. Frequent colds and flus, cancer, cardiovascular diseases, arthritis, and allergies are all consequences of congestive disorders. These medical problems may be prevented or treated through a process of cleansing, fasting, and detoxification. These represent different degrees of a process which reduces toxin intake and enhances toxin elimination.

All of the programs contained in this book combine aspects of these fasting and detoxification processes. I have written specific programs for dealing with sugar, nicotine, alcohol, and caffeine, and chemicals (drugs)—what I call SNACCs. In each program, I discuss the physiologic actions and reactions involved, the hazards and ill effects of each substance, and methods for handling and clearing these adverse habits.

The beginning of the process for healing our abuses requires motivation from within to change unwanted habits. This often requires us to address the underlying emotions which may perpetuate the problem. Then we must create a workable plan and gather our will power to begin. The Detox Diet discussed throughout this book alkalinizes the body, helps us feel better quickly, and lessens feelings of withdrawal. Water, exercise, and vitamin and mineral supplements also support the detoxification process.

I work with three primary tenets of naturopathy, adapted from Jim Sharp's book, *Basic Principles of Total Health—Harmonious Integration of Body Mind and Spirit:*
1. The primary cause of disease is the accumulation of unnecessary wastes which are not properly eliminated, resulting in poison retention and subsequent disease.
2. Your body is designed to support optimal function. Listen to its signals.
3. Given the proper environment, your body has the power to heal itself and return to its normal healthy state.

I believe that patients and physicians alike should be oriented to live and practice with a commonsense approach that first looks at lifestyle as a place to promote rejuvenation, then to natural therapies, and finally to pharmaceutical drugs and surgery. Lifestyle factors include diet, exercise, stress management, and attitudes. Natural therapies include supplements, herbs, homeopathics, and hands-on healing such as massage, osteopathy, and chiropractic. Pharmaceutical drugs or surgery are appropriate when a situation is acute or severe, or if natural therapies are not working.

Put simply, the key to maintaining metabolic balance is to maximize nutrition and to eliminate toxins.

My goal is to place your health and that of your family back into your own hands. In fact, so much of your health is up to you. Take the initiative to do what you can to be vital and healthy. It is really worth it!

Be clean and clear, healthy and free,

Elson M. Haas, MD.

CHAPTER ONE

Gastrointestinal Tract Health

Gastrointestinal function and ecology is at the core of human health. Imbalances can affect overall well-being. Likewise, the structure and functions of the intestines determine total body toxin load and are essential to the process of detoxification. Cleansing and healing the GI tract (especially the colon) provides a base for effective detoxification.

"We are what we eat and assimilate, and not what we eliminate," is really saying that our GI tract function is vital to the process of nourishing our body and controlling toxicity through elimination, a process which truly begins in the colon. Furthermore, we must regularly cleanse the intestinal system to effectively detoxify the body. Specific therapies are discussed throughout this book; in this chapter, I want to provide a basic discussion of the GI tract process and its contribution to overall health—a relationship often overlooked in Western medicine.

SOME IMPRESSIVE GI TRACT FACTS

- The total GI mucosal surface is made up of many microscopic crypts and crevices, most of which are in the small intestine and have the interactive area equivalent to the size of a tennis court.

- There are more bacteria (10^{12}) in a gram of stool than there are stars in the known universe.

- The microbes of the GI tract constitute a very metabolically active area of the body, second only to the liver.

- The total weight of the bacteria located in the colon of the average human equals approximately five pounds (or about the weight of our liver).

- The digestive organs manufacture nearly a gallon of juices per day to help digest and utilize the food we eat.

In this model (which I call Functional Integrated Medicine), the function, ecology, and permeability of the GI tract are crucial to the health of each patient. Dysbiosis is the term used to describe imbalance of GI function (specifically, incomplete food digestion and assimilation) or its microbial populations. Preventive medicine works with the theory that abnormal function precedes pathology, and hence the GI tract is assessed for dysbiosis. Therefore, to prevent pathology, normal functioning, specifically of the GI tract, must be restored. If this concept of prevention is incorporated into mainstream medicine, we can keep people healthier longer and prevent disease by evaluating and maintaining proper internal function and environment. Fortunately, this shift in thinking is picking up speed around the country.

The GI tract is composed of the mouth and teeth, the esophagus and stomach, the small intestine (duodenum, jejunum, and ileum) and large intestine (colon). Its proper function begins with **adequate chewing**, which is essential for good nutrition and health. Other digestive organs include the salivary glands, pancreas, gall bladder, GI mucous glands, and liver. Salivary enzymes begin digestion and the process is continued by stomach hydrochloric acid and enzymes, plus the many pancreatic enzymes which are released into the upper small intestine. Finally, the gall bladder releases bile to promote fat digestion. Assimilation of most nutrients occurs in the small intestine; the colon absorbs water, bile salts, and a few other substances in order to prepare the remainder of the colonic contents for elimination.

Regular elimination is also crucial to overall health and control of the level of toxicity in the body—constipation is actually a greater problem than most doctors and patients realize. Hydration, diet, level of physical activity, and stress all affect our eliminative function.

Health and proper functional integrity of the huge mucosal membrane surface area of the GI tract allows the proper assimilation of nutrients. Even minor disruptions such as inflammation or infection may cause abnormal absorption and increased barrier permeability. With increased intestinal permeability, absorption goes out of balance and larger-than-normal molecules get absorbed which can cause allergic reactions and other abnormal immune responses. There is a delicate balance between the assimilation of needed nutrients and the exclusion of toxic substances. Abnormal organisms within the intestinal lumen may produce toxins which can significantly affect mental and physical health. Also, certain pathogens within the GI tract may generate autoimmune reactions in the particularly vulnerable environment of the small bowel, where the majority of our immune cells are located.

Problems of dysbiosis, abnormal GI mucosal permeability, infection, and inflammation are exceedingly common and may cause both gastrointestinal complaints and other health concerns. The GI tract is stressed and otherwise adversely affected by:

- refined foods and sugar
- excess fatty and rich foods
- overeating and failing to chew more than once or twice per mouthful of food
- drinking too much with meals, thus diluting our digestive juices and reducing our ability to properly break down food
- food chemicals, pesticides, and environmental toxins
- the persistent use of alcohol, caffeine, and nicotine
- use of prescription, over-the-counter, and recreational drugs
- lack of fiber and whole foods, specifically lacking fresh fruits, vegetables, whole grains, and legumes in the diet

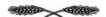

The GI tract is especially sensitive to emotional turmoil. A stressful lifestyle may adversely affect motility, digestive enzyme output, and overall function. Over 30 gut hormones have been identified, many of which also act as neurotransmitters. Chemical exposure (specifically ingested chemicals), travel and subsequent parasitic infections, or the overuse of antibiotics can cause intestinal dysfunction and disease. It may take years for the gut to recover from this kind of damage.

It is also important to maintain proper levels of friendly bacteria within the colon and make sure that their numbers decrease in concentration when progressing up the GI tract into the small intestine or stomach. Overgrowth of abnormal bacteria, fermenting yeasts, and parasites can disturb GI function causing inflammation along the sensitive mucous membrane of the GI tract and thereby adversely affecting the assimilation of food and nutrients.

Abnormal permeability, often called "leaky gut," creates GI imbalance which can lead to systemic disease. Over-assimilation of non-nutrient compounds and under-assimilation of required nutrients may produce deficiencies, as well as allergies and other immune system problems. Inflammation or infection in the GI tract, food allergies, and the overuse of alcohol and non-steroid anti-inflammatory drugs (NSAIDs) can all cause problems in permeability. Disorders such as irritable bowel syndrome, Crohn's disease, rheumatoid arthritis, and HIV infections are frequently associated with leaky gut and permeability problems. A common condition involves fermentation from yeast overgrowth, specifically *Candida albicans* and other related Candida species, which can lead to a large variety of symptoms and which are often associated with permeability problems.

There are literally billions of microorganisms inhabiting the healthy GI tract. Friendly ones include E. Coli (the bacteria *Escherichia coli*), various streptococci, and *Lactobacillus acidophilus,* as well as *Lactobacillus bifidis (Bifidobacteria),* which is predominant in infants and children. However, many other undesirable organisms reside in the GI tract, particularly in the large intestine. These can include yeasts, abnormal bacteria such as Klebsiella (not always pathogenic) and Citrobacter species, a variety of pathogenic parasites that include *Giardia lamblia* and *Blastocystis hominis,* and amoebas such as *histolytica, hartmani,* and *coli.*

HEALING THE GI TRACT

An effective way to think about and heal the gastrointestinal tract has been developed and taught by Jeff Bland, Ph.D., in his nutritional education seminars. It is part of an approach to health care he calls *Functional Medicine.* Preventive medicine focuses on basic functions within the body, balancing or rebalancing them when they are not right through the use of supportive nutrients and appropriate natural substances. This is similar to *OrthoMolecular Medicine,* a concept coined by Linus Pauling with whom Dr. Bland worked for a number of years. Currently, Dr. Bland and his team at *HealthComm* in Gig Harbor, Washington, are working to find better ways to assess, heal, and support GI anatomy and physiology, as a way to remedy illness and generate health.

There have been a number of new tests developed in the last decade which look at digestion and assimilation, GI mucosal surface health, and the presence or absence of appropriate or pathogenic bacteria, yeasts, and parasites. Several licensed laboratories across the country (particularly Great Smokies Diagnostic Lab in Asheville, North Carolina) have led the way in developing very useful, clinically significant tests, which follow.

GASTROINTESTINAL TESTS

Allopathic Medical Tests

1) Upper GI, or the Barium Swallow, X-Ray Study

A series of x-rays is taken (viewed with dye) from the mouth to the small intestine. It is useful for identifying anatomical and motility problems as it detects significant problems like gastric or peptic ulcers, hiatal hernias, and tumors within (or pushing into) the upper GI tract. Concerns with this test and the barium enema include the x-ray exposure, constipation from the relatively nontoxic dye (which only rarely causes reactions), and fluid/nutrient imbalance resulting from the enemas and oral purgatives used in preparation for these tests. Cleansing the bowels after the tests by drinking water and taking vitamin C will help counter some of the radiation and toxin exposure.

2) The Barium Enema

This rather unpleasant test involves the slow injection of a highly pressurized enema into a cleaned-out colon to examine the area from rectum to small intestine. It is used to diagnose ulcerative colitis in progressed stages, tumors (both benign and cancerous), and misshapen colons, which are often the result of many years of poor diet and constipation.

3) Gastroscopes and Colonoscopes (also Sigmoidoscopes)

The gastroscope is a fiberoptic tube that is inserted through the mouth to view the esophagus, stomach, and pyloric area. The colonoscope is inserted through the anus and travels around the colon. Both scopes are used to search out inflammation, polyps, tumors, or ulcers. A less comprehensive test employs the "silver tube" or sigmoidoscope—a rigid instrument used to assess the rectum and sigmoid colon only. The obvious advantage of the scopes for testing is the total avoidance of any exposure to radiation. Biopsies or even complete excisions can be performed utilizing the instruments, often avoiding, or at least postponing, more invasive surgery. These procedures can, however, be quite painful, and doctors often give multiple antipain and tranquilizing drugs, or even general anesthesia from which it may take several days to recover.

Functional GI Tests

4) CDSA—Comprehensive Digestive Stool Analysis

This simple assessment has been a medical breakthrough. A stool is collected and mailed overnight to a lab where it is evaluated for digestion of animal proteins, vegetable matter, starch, and fatty acids. Stool pH, intestinal immune function (with the addition of secretory Immunoglobulin A), and the presence of mucus, blood, and certain enzymes are also measured. Culturing is done to locate both normal and abnormal bacteria and yeast or fungus. If any abnormal organisms are detected, sensitivity testing is done with both natural substances (such as garlic, grapefruit seed extract, caprylic acid) and pharmaceutical agents (such as antibiotics and antifungals) to determine which agents kill or inhibit the growth of the detected organism. This allows the practitioner and patient to select the right treatment for their particular condition. This information then gives us a therapy that involves the **removal** of abnormal organisms, **replacement** of diminished enzymes or hydrochloric acid, **reinoculation** with appropriate helpful microorganisms (probiotics), and **repair** of the GI mucosa. This constitutes the 4R program, which is discussed later in this chapter as "the 5R program," with the addition of **rebalancing** diet and lifestyle. There are no side effects or medical concerns with the CDSA or the Parasite Study other than the psychological discomfort that some people experience from having to handle their own feces.

5) Parasite Study

Certain laboratories specialize in identifying parasitic infections through stool exams. These exams require a loose or a special "purged" stool collection—a watery sample that is observed under a special microscope. (The purging process may cause some diarrhea, but its mildly cleansing effect may have some benefit as well.) These parasitic infections are quite common, even in people who do not travel outside the United States. The lab I currently use is the Institute for Parasitic Diseases (IPD) in Phoenix, Arizona; their findings correlate well with clinical symptoms. I look for parasites in anyone who presents with GI dysfunction (especially pain, gas, bloating, and nausea), allergies, fatigue, insomnia, teeth grinding at night, anxiety, or other psycho-emotional symptoms.

6) Intestinal Permeability

This is a simple test that measures the small intestine's ability to absorb needed nutrients and discriminate against harmful substances. After drinking a solution comprised of two sugars (lactulose and mannitol), a urine sample is collected and the levels of these two sugars are measured. Mannitol is normally absorbed at approximately 20%, while lactulose should be absorbed very little, if at all. People with increased intestinal permeability absorb excess lactulose. This suggests that they also inappropriately absorb other larger molecules due to damaged intestinal walls. Such absorption can cause secondary immunologic reactions and subsequent food allergies and intolerance. Working the 5R program will often normalize intestinal permeability. This test and the Breath Test have no side effects at all. The two mostly non-absorbable sugars mentioned above occasionally cause temporarily loose bowels.

7) Breath Test for Small Intestine Bacterial Overgrowth

This test measures levels of hydrogen and methane gases in breath samples to assess bacterial overgrowth in the small intestine. Although this problem is more common in the elderly, it should be considered for anyone with gas, bloating, diarrhea, or carbohydrate intolerance. Bacterial overgrowth can compromise health both in the GI tract and throughout the body and can lead to malabsorption, failure to thrive, anemia, weakened immunity, and increased risk of colon cancer (intestinal bacteria may produce additional carcinogens). This test is suggested when the standard 5R approach is not working effectively enough.

8) Detoxification Profile

This is a relatively new procedure that tests the detoxification functions of the liver. Our body must be able to metabolize and clear xenobiotics (environmental chemicals), endotoxins (generated from gut flora), and our own biochemicals (including hormones and cholesterol). The Detoxification Profile measures two primary liver pathways: Phase I (oxidation and reduction, such as in caffeine metabolism) and Phase II (glycine, glutathione, and sulfate conjugation, as well as glucuronidation). Each demonstrates the patient's ability or inability to detoxify certain types of chemicals. Test doses of caffeine, aspirin, and acetaminophen are given and then both salivary and urine samples are taken and studied to identify the level of detoxification. The only concern with this test would be any adverse reactions to the testing agents.

I use these tests judiciously whenever I see a patient with gastrointestinal concerns or systemic symptoms correlated with gastrointestinal dysbiosis, inflammation, or toxicity. After gathering information from these tests, I decide upon a course of therapy which is often interdisciplinary in its approach. Detoxification practices—the focus of this book—are an important first step in healing, since many diseases are related to congestion and toxicity from overintake and improper elimination.

A therapeutic regimen often includes dietary changes such as avoiding certain foods or food groups and adding more fresh, high-fiber and low-fat fruits, vegetables, and whole grains. I also address abusive habits and try to motivate my patients to give this therapy a fair chance. Most modern-day abuses—Sugar, Nicotine, Alcohol, Caffeine, and Chemicals—are psychoactive substances which have mental and emotional effects. I believe that giving up at least the habitual use of these SNACCs (as I call them) is extremely important. I also promote chewing your food thoroughly along with regular and systematic undereating. If we make what we eat wholesome and nourishing, we will not only add years to our lives, but life to our years. Choosing the right foods and diet for ourselves, our activity level, and the climate in which we live is the key.

Other lifestyle and therapeutic activities for GI health include:

1. **Learning to manage stress.** Our sensitive digestive tract works better when we are calm.

2. **Setting up an exercise program.** Exercise improves digestive functions, stimulates lymphatic flow, and supports immune function.

3. **Applying musculoskeletal therapies.** This may involve osteopathic or chiropractic realignment of the spine and massage.

4. **Using nutritional supplements and herbs.**

5. **Seeking professional advice on the use of pharmaceutical (or herbal) agents** to remove infectious and harmful organisms, including abnormal bacteria, yeasts, and parasites.

The 5R Plan

Let me now review the 5R Gastrointestinal Support Plan. This progressive therapeutic program normalizes the function, environment, and tissue health of the GI tract and must be tailored to the individual according to his or her particular evaluation. The five steps are:

1) **Rebalance**—your diet, your lifestyle, and your life. (This "R" added to Dr. Bland's 4R Plan by my associate, Scott V. Anderson, M.D.) This is important as these areas contribute to health and the state of the digestive tract. Staying away from sugar, refined foods, and irritating substances such as caffeine and alcohol can make a big difference. Learning to deal with stress and developing coping and relaxation skills can help calm the GI tract and support better digestion and assimilation.

Changing habits is not easy. A nutritional counselor, psychologist, or hypnotherapist can help by making us aware of the way old conditioning undermines our new positive health habits.

2) **Remove**—any offending organisms, particularly pathogenic microflora and/or any food antigens that cause allergic and immunologic reactions.

At this therapeutic level, we evaluate and treat any organisms that do not belong in the human GI tract. These include *Giardia lamblia*, abnormal types or levels of yeast organisms such as *Candida albicans,* and bacterial pathogens. Sensitivity testing (finding what therapeutic agents eliminate the specific microbe) can be done on most of these organisms to find the appropriate pharmaceutical or natural medications. Often, there is more than one type of pathogen, and a combination of medications may be needed. Treatments will vary according to the practitioner's training. One useful book is *Guess What Came to Dinner* by Ann Louise Gittleman; the author discusses the great prevalence of parasitic disease and the best ways, both natural and pharmaceutical, to treat each specific parasite.

We also encourage following an elimination diet that avoids allergenic foods and removes irritating substances such as caffeine, alcohol, refined sugar, and flour. Following a "hypoallergenic" diet involves eliminating common food allergens such as cow's milk, eggs, gluten grains (wheat, rye, barley, and oats), chocolate, coffee, and peanuts. Any food that is consumed regularly or over-consumed should also be eliminated. A diet of fruits, vegetables, rice and beans, fish, and poultry is usually an improvement for most people, producing a reduction of symptoms and an increase in energy.

3) **Replace**—inadequate amounts of hydrochloric acid (HCl), digestive enzymes, and pancreatic products. Fiber supplementation may also be necessary.

Nutritional substances in this category aid in food breakdown and in its subsequent absorption into the bloodstream for travel to the metabolic factory of the liver. Proper digestion reduces the allergenic and inflammatory effects that occur from larger, more complex molecules.

The CDSA (Comprehensive Digestive Stool Analysis) helps identify digestion weaknesses and guides the practitioner and patient toward the proper replacement support. For instance, enzyme or hydrochloric acid insufficiency is common in people who experience indigestion, gas and bloating, belching and flatulence, and the presence of food particles in the stool. Yeast overgrowth is another problem, and should be ruled out prior to treatment.

Replacement products are categorized as follows:

- Betaine and other forms of HCl
- Plant-derived digestive enzymes (proteases, amylases, lipases, and cellulases)
- Animal-derived enzymes (proteases, amylases, lipases, and elastases)
- Microbe-derived digestive enzymes
- Lactase enzyme supplements
- Fiber, both soluble and insoluble

4) **Reinoculation**—refers to the reintroduction or "reflorastation" of desirable bacterial flora as well as special nutrients such as fructooligosaccharides (FOS) which support the growth and function of friendly microorganisms.

Reinoculation includes supplementation of symbiotic bacteria normally present in the healthy GI tract. These bacteria, called "probiotics," include *Lactobacillus acidophilus* (also *bulgaricus* and *thermophilus*) and *Bifidobacteria bifidus*, (also *longum, infantis,* and *breve*). They are predominant in the gut of young, healthy people but often decrease with age, especially with the use of antibiotics, exposure to toxic chemicals and metals, and with substance abuse (particularly alcohol and caffeine). Also, recurrent infections (including GI pathogenic and parasitic infections), abnormal intestinal pH, lowered immune status, and abnormal digestion may contribute to imbalanced flora.

A second CDSA can determine whether or not this reflorastation has been successful. The supplements used should be viable strains of the microbes stated above and should be stored and shipped at cool temperatures. Probiotics are available primarily in powder form and as capsules or tablets, although cultured yogurt or milk products also contain some Lactobacilli species.

5) **Repair**—means providing nutritional support for the regeneration and healing of the gastrointestinal lining and is probably the most important component of the 5R Program.

The GI mucosal cells represent the largest mass of biochemically active and proliferating cells in the body. Repair is needed when the structure or function of the gastrointestinal mucosa loses its integrity. Both the CDSA and Permeability tests will help identify disrepair or dysbiosis. Loss of integrity can result from infection (particularly from parasites or yeast), food allergy, chronic nutritional deficiency, chemical exposure, inflammatory bowel disease, and general dysbiosis.

I believe that proper detoxification begins with understanding gastrointestinal function and its affect on overall health. You will find that these guidelines, when combined with regular exercise, will improve your health, vitality, and the functioning of your gastrointestinal tract. This, in turn, reduces the chance of degenerative and chronic diseases, and helps slow the aging process. Remember, prevention is the key!

Some of the important nutrients for healing the GI tract include the amino acid L-glutamine, pantothenic acid, zinc, vitamin A, antioxidants (such as vitamins C and E, beta-carotene, and selenium), the bioflavonoid quercitin, essential fatty acids, inulin, and fiber (particularly the soluble kind). Herbs such as aloe vera, licorice root, and comfrey root also have positive healing effects on the mucosal lining of the gastrointestinal tract. These nutrients play a key role in GI mucosal cell differentiation, growth, function, and repair. The following chart describes these important nutrients.

NUTRIENTS FOR HEALING THE GI TRACT

1) **L-glutamine** is a nonessential amino acid used as fuel by active cells, particularly the enterocytes of the GI tract. Extra L-glutamine is needed to heal the GI tract during disease.

2) **Pantothenic Acid (vitamin B$_5$)** is necessary for protein synthesis and ATP energy production, both of which are involved in the tissue healing process. It is also works with vitamin C to handle stress and support the adrenals.

3) **Ascorbic Acid (vitamin C)** is essential for collagen formation, which is the basis for connective tissue repair, wound healing, and general tissue strength. It also works as an antioxidant to counter free radicals which can damage and inflame tissues.

4) **Vitamin A (retinol)** and **Beta-Carotene**, the nontoxic precursor of vitamin A, is needed for normal growth, function, and repair of epithelial cells, including those in the GI mucosa. Taking both nutrients ensures proper levels of vitamin A.

5) **Vitamin E** is an essential antioxidant which defends cell membrane integrity and function, thus helping to protect active enzyme systems within the cells.

6) **Zinc (picolinate, as one bioavailable example)** is essential to tissue health and repair, enzyme function, maintaining the integrity of the cell membrane structure, and cell replication. All of these processes are needed for the function and repair of the GI lining. Recent research from France indicates that zinc can be unusually effective in healing GI tissue inflammation.

7) **Selenium** is an important antioxidant for chemical detoxification, which protects GI tract cells from damage and allows appropriate repair.

8) **Quercitin** is a bioflavonoid with antihistamine and anti-inflammatory effects, useful in reducing food allergy reactions and helping in tissue repair.

9) **Essential Fatty Acids (EFAs)** help to maintain the integrity of cell membranes and protect and heal the cells and tissues. Good sources include flax seed oil, fish oils (EPA and DHA), and cold pressed, unheated vegetable oils.

10) **Inulin** is a storage carbohydrate found in onions and Jerusalem artichokes that acts as fuel for colon epithelial cells and promotes healing and energy generation.

11) **Aloe Vera,** in its purified and extracted juice form, is both soothing and healing to the GI tract mucosa and tissue.

12) **Licorice Root** and **DGL (deglycirrhized licorice)** has an anti-inflammatory effect in the GI tract. DGL is particularly helpful in healing ulcers and other stomach inflammations.

13) **Comfrey Root** soothes and heals the gastrointestinal mucosa.*

14) **Glutathione, L-cysteine,** and **N-acetylcysteine** provide fuel and act as protective antioxidants and detoxification supporters for the GI mucosa and cellular enzyme systems.

15) **Fiber,** especially the soluble type, protects and promotes proper movement of feces through the GI tract without irritation. Insoluble fiber may also help lessen gut toxicity.

16) **FOS (fructooligosaccharides)** fuels colon bacteria and protects colon cells from pathogenic infections. Some yeast and bacterial strains use FOS as a food source; therefore, it is important to remove or reduce these microbial populations before adding FOS.

17) **Calories** from fresh fruits and vegetables, whole grains, seeds, and legumes are needed to repair damaged or inflamed tissues and maintain energy levels during the GI tract healing program.

* There is some concern about toxicity from excessive use of comfrey root, however small amounts over a limited period of time should be safe and helpful.

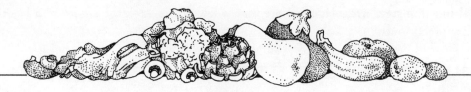

IMPORTANT ELEMENTS OF HEALTHY EATING

- Eat whole foods, particularly fresh fruits, vegetables, whole grains, and vegetable proteins (legumes, nuts, and seeds).

- We are what we eat—put only quality food into your body. Reduce refined foods, sugar, excess fatty and rich foods, and foods with additives or synthetic coloring.

- Drink no more than 4 oz. of liquids with meals, as it can dilute the digestive juices.

- Chew your food thoroughly, eat in a relaxed environment, and never eat when upset.

- Get sufficient fiber in your diet by eating the majority of your foods from item #1 above and/or by taking additional psyllium husk and flaxseed meal.

- Drink 6 to 8 glasses of water daily, plus herbal teas.

- Use nutritional supplements and herbs as appropriate. Supplement your digestive function as needed with hydrochloric acid, digestive enzymes, and pancreatic products.

- Moderate your use of alcohol, caffeine and nicotine. Beware of excessive use of prescription, OTC, and recreational drugs.

- Exercise. If you don't yet have an exercise program, set one up. Do it regularly and with the right combination of activities that will provide strength, flexibility, endurance, and enjoyment.

- Maintain regular elimination. Your diet, exercise and stress levels should allow your bowels to move at least once or twice daily. After illness or antibiotic use, replace friendly GI flora by taking probiotics (acidophilus and other positive digestive bacteria). If this is not sufficient to restore normal digestion and elimination, and your GI function stays irregular for more than a few weeks, seek the advice of a health-care practitioner.

CHAPTER TWO

General Detoxification and Cleansing

◆

Toxicity has become a great concern in the twentieth century and I predict that the process of detoxification will be an important tool for twenty-first century medicine. Threatening our health are powerful chemicals, air and water pollution, radiation, and nuclear waste. We ingest new chemicals, use more drugs, eat more sugary and refined foods, and abuse ourselves daily with stimulants and/or sedatives. Cancer and cardiovascular disease are on the rise; arthritis, allergies, obesity, and skin problems are also rapidly increasing; and a wide range of symptoms such as headaches, fatigue, pains, coughs, gastrointestinal problems, immune weaknesses, sexual diseases, and psychological distress are being seen by physicians in record numbers. Although a connection between increased toxicity and increases in diseases is obvious, it is important to understand how it occurs so that we may avoid or eliminate it from our lives.

Toxicity occurs on two basic bodily levels—external and internal. We can acquire toxins from our environment by breathing them, by ingesting them, or through physical contact with them. Most drugs, food additives, and allergens can create toxic elements in the body. In fact, any substance can become toxic when used in excess.

Internally, our body produces toxins through normal everyday functions. Biochemical and cellular activities generate substances that need to be eliminated. These unstable molecules, called *free radicals*, are biochemical toxins and are considered a common factor in chronic disease. When these biochemical toxins are not counteracted or eliminated, they can irritate or inflame the cells and tissues, blocking normal functions on all levels of the body. Microbes such as intestinal bacteria, foreign bacteria, yeasts, and parasites produce metabolic waste products that we must handle. Even our thoughts, emotions, and stress can increase biochemical toxicity. The proper elimination of these toxins is essential. Clearly, the healthy human body can handle certain levels of toxins; **the concern is with excess intake or production of toxins or a reduction in the elimination processes.**

A toxin is basically any substance that creates irritating and/or harmful effects in the body, undermining our health and stressing our biochemical or organ functions. This irritation may result from the side effects of pharmaceutical drugs or from unusual physiological patterns. The irritating chemicals or free radicals in recreational drugs can also cause tissue degeneration. Negative "ethers," psychic or spiritual influences, bad relationships, thought patterns, and emotions can have toxic effects on the body.

Toxicity occurs when we ingest more than we can utilize and eliminate. Homeostasis refers to balanced bodily functions. This balance is disturbed when we feed ourselves more than we need or when we abuse specific substances. Toxicity may depend on the dosage, frequency, or potency of the toxin. A toxin may produce an immediate or rapid onset of symptoms, as many pesticides and some drugs do, or it may have long-term effects, as when asbestos exposure leads to lung cancer.

If our body is working well, with good immune and eliminative functions, it can handle everyday exposure to toxins. The purpose of this chapter is to discuss ways to support the elimination of excessive toxins, mucus, congestion, and disease and to prevent the buildup of further toxicity. The cleansing process encourages our immune system to handle the elimination of toxins and abnormal cells generated by the body.

OUR GENERAL DETOXIFICATION SYSTEMS

Gastrointestinal—liver, gallbladder, colon, and the whole GI tract

Urinary—kidneys, bladder, and urethra

Respiratory—lungs, bronchial tubes, throat, sinuses, and nose

Lymphatic—lymph channels and lymph nodes

Skin and dermal—sweat and sebaceous glands and tears

Our body handles toxins either by neutralizing, transforming, or eliminating them. For example, many of the antioxidant nutrients, such as vitamins C and E, beta-carotene, zinc, and selenium may neutralize free-radical molecules. The liver helps transform many toxic substances into harmless agents, which the blood carries away to the kidneys; the liver also sends wastes through the bile into the intestines, where it is eliminated. We also clear toxins by sweating, either from exercise or heat; our sinuses expel excess mucus when congested; and our skin releases toxins as skin rashes.

Mental detoxification is also important. Cleansing our minds of negative thought patterns is essential to health, and physical detoxification can aid this process. Emotionally, detoxification helps us uncover and express hidden frustrations, anger, resentments, and fear, and replace them with forgiveness, love, joy, and hope. Many people experience new clarity of purpose in life during cleansing processes. A light detoxification over a couple of days can help us feel better; a longer process and deeper commitment to eliminating certain abusive habits and eating a better diet can help us change our whole life. Detoxification is part of a transformational medicine that instills change at many levels. Change and evolution are keys to healing.

I want to express some concerns about overelimination or overdetoxification, which I occasionally see. Some people go to extremes with fasting, laxatives, enemas, colonics, diuretics, and even exercise and begin to lose essential nutrients from their body. This can cause protein or vitamin-mineral deficiencies. So, although congestion from overintake and underelimination is a more common problem in this culture, excessive detoxification can be equally harmful.

WHO Should Detoxify?

Almost everyone needs to detox and rest their body from time to time. Some of us need to cleanse more frequently or work more continually to rebalance our body. *Cleansing* or detoxification is but one part of the trilogy of nutritional action (the others being *building*, or toning, and *balancing*, or maintenance). A regular, balanced diet devoid of excess necessitates less intensive detoxification. Our body has a daily elimination cycle, mostly carried out at night and in the early morning up until breakfast. When we eat a congesting diet higher in fats, meats, dairy products, refined foods, and chemicals, detoxification becomes more important, particularly to those who eat excessively, and to those who eat excessively at night.

Our individual lifestyle provides clues for deciding how and when to detoxify. If we have any symptoms or diseases of toxicity and congestion, we will likely benefit from detoxification practices. It is like a vacation for our body and digestive tract.

Common toxicity symptoms include headache, fatigue, congestion, backaches, aching or swollen joints, digestive problems, "allergy" symptoms, and sensitivity to environmental agents such as chemicals, perfumes, and synthetics. Dietary changes or avoidance of the symptom-causing agents is usually beneficial. However, it is important to differentiate between allergic and toxicity symptoms in order to determine the appropriate medical care. This detox program, fasting, and juice cleansing can be genuinely helpful in reducing allergy symptoms; however, allergies present a dynamic subtly different from toxicity.

SIGNS AND SYMPTOMS OF TOXICITY		
Headaches	Frequent colds*	Mood changes*
Joint pains	Irritated eyes	Anxiety
Coughs	Immune weakness*	Depression*
Wheezing	Environmental sensitivity	Fatigue*
Sore throat	Sinus congestion	Skin rashes*
Tight or stiff neck	Fever	Hives
Angina pectoris	Runny nose	Nausea
Circulatory deficits	Nervousness	Indigestion
High blood fats	Sleepiness*	Anorexia
Backaches	Insomnia*	Bad breath
Itchy nose	Dizziness*	Constipation

* These symptoms could also result from deficiency.

Detoxification and cleansing can contribute to the healing of many acute and chronic illnesses that result from short- or long-term congestive patterns. Detox and cleansing benefits people with addictions to numerous substances. However, because withdrawal symptoms can commonly occur with the detoxification of many drugs, I recommend conscious, informed management of the detox process.

Detoxification is also an important component in treating obesity. Many of the toxins we ingest or make are stored in the fatty tissues; hence, obesity is almost always associated with toxicity. When we lose weight, we reduce our body fat and thereby our toxic load. However, during weight loss we also release more toxins and need to protect ourselves from nutrient depletion through extra supplementation, including taking additional antioxidants to balance these toxins. Exercise will also promote the loss of excess pounds and help further detoxification.

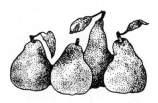

PROBLEMS RELATED TO CONGESTION / STAGNATION / TOXICITY		
Acne	Gout	Stroke
Abscesses	Obesity	Prostate disease
Boils	Infections by:	Menstrual problems
Eczema	Bacteria	Vaginitis
Allergies	Virus	Varicose veins
Arthritis	Fungus	Diabetes
Asthma	Parasites	Peptic ulcers
Constipation	Worms	Gastritis
Colitis	Uterine fibroid tumors	Pancreatitis
Hemorrhoids	Cancer	Mental illness
Diverticulitis	Cataracts	Multiple sclerosis
Cirrhosis	Colds	Alzheimer's disease
Hepatitis	Bronchitis	Senility
Fibrocystic breast disease	Pneumonia	Parkinson's disease
Atherosclerosis	Sinusitis	Drug addiction
Heart disease	Emphysema	Tension headaches
Hypertension	Kidney stones	Migraine headaches
Thrombophlebitis	Kidney disease	Gallstones

Of course, not all of these problems are related solely to toxicity nor will they be completely cured by detoxification. Still, many conditions are created by nutritional abuses and can be alleviated by eliminating the related toxins and following this program.

WHAT Is Detoxification?

Detoxification is the process of either clearing toxins from the body or neutralizing or transforming them, and hence clearing excess mucus and congestion. Fats (especially oxidized fats and cholesterol), free radicals, and other irritating molecules act as toxins on an internal level. Functionally, poor digestion, colon sluggishness and dysfunction, reduced liver function, and poor elimination through the kidneys, respiratory tract, and skin all increase toxicity.

Detoxification involves dietary and lifestyle changes that reduce the intake of toxins while improving elimination. The avoidance of chemicals from food or other sources, including refined food, sugar, caffeine, alcohol, tobacco, and drugs, helps minimize the toxin load. Drinking extra water (purified) and increasing fiber by including more fruits and vegetables in the diet are also essential steps. Moving to a less congesting diet, as shown in the accompanying table, will also induce healing.

DETOXIFICATION RANGE						
Most Congesting ◄—					—► *Least Congesting*	
drugs	fats	sweets	nuts	rice	roots	fruits
allergenic foods	fried foods	milk	seeds	millet	squashes	greens
organ meats	refined flour	eggs	beans	buckwheat	other vegetables	herbs
hydrogenated fats	meats	baked goods	oats	pasta		water
			wheat	potatoes		
More Potentially Toxic ◄—				—► *More Detoxifying*		

Detoxification therapy—particularly fasting—is the oldest known medical treatment on earth and a completely natural process. Of the thousands of people I know who have used cleansing programs, the vast majority have experienced very positive results. I believe this detoxification process to be a lay therapy for medicine in the 21st century and an important first step toward healing our planet.

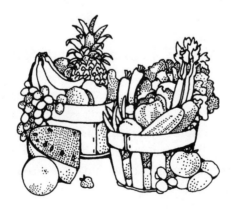

WHEN Is the Best Time to Detoxify?

Whenever we feel congested, our first step is to follow detoxification procedures fine-tuned to our specific needs. I have found that when I start to feel congested from too much food, people, or activities, I will feel better if I can exercise, sauna or steam, drink loads of fluids, eat lightly, take vitamins C and A, and get a good night's sleep. If I feel my colon requires further cleansing, I take stimulating herbs.

Our bodies have natural cleansing cycles when they want a lighter diet, more liquids, and greater elimination than intake. This occurs daily (usually from the night until midmorning, about an hour after we wake) and it may occur weekly and more commonly for a few days a month. Women, in particular, are aware of this natural cleansing time with their menstrual cycle. In fact, many women feel better both premenstrually and during their periods if they follow a simple cleansing program of more juices, greens, lighter foods, and herbs.

To summarize, *seasonal changes* are key times of stress when we need to reduce our outer demands and consumptions and listen to the way our inner world mirrors the natural cycles. **Spring** is the key time for detoxification; **autumn** is also important. I suggest at least a one- to two-week program at these times. In spring, we may eat more citrus fruits, fresh greens, juices, or the Master Cleanser lemonade diet (p. 119); while in autumn we may dine on harvest fruits, such as apples or grapes, and seasonal vegetables. An abundance of fresh fruits and vegetables are appropriate for **summer**; and whole grains, legumes, vegetables, and soups best simplify our diet in **winter.**

The sample yearly program provided here is designed for a basically healthy person who eats well. It is not appropriate for people with heart problems, extreme fatigue, underweight conditions, or poor circulation (those who experience coldness). More complete, in-depth fasting programs may release even greater amounts of toxins (see Chapter 10: Fasting and Juice Cleansing). Releasing too much toxicity can make sick people sicker; if this happens, they need to increase fluids and eat normally again until they feel better. People with cancer need to be very careful about how they detoxify, and often they need regular, quality nourishment. Fasting should be done only under the care of an experienced physician. All people should avoid fasting just prior to surgery, and should wait four to six weeks before detoxifying after it. Pregnant or lactating women should avoid heavy detoxification, though they can usually handle mild programs, which should be undertaken only with the guidance of a qualified practitioner.

SAMPLE YEAR-LONG DETOX PROGRAM

~ SPRING ~

For 7–21 days between March 10 and April 15, use one or more of the following plans:

- Master Cleanser (lemonade diet, see p. 119).
- Fruits, vegetables, greens.
- Juices of fruits, vegetables, and greens.
- Herbs with any of the above.
- These plans can be alternated, or can include a 3–5 day supervised water fast.
- Remember to take time for the transition back to the regular diet (about half as long as the fast itself), which hopefully will have changed for the better.
- Elimination and food testing can also be done at this time.

~ MID-SPRING ~

Take a 3-day cleanse around mid May as a reminder of healthy habits and as an enhancer of food awareness.

~ SUMMER ~

Try one week of fruits and vegetables and/or fresh juices to usher in the warm weather sometime between June 10 and July 4.

~ LATE SUMMER ~

Take a 3-day cleanse of fruit and vegetable juices around mid to late August.

~ AUTUMN ~

Take a 7–10 day cleanse between September 11 and October 5, such as:

- Grape fast—whole and juiced—all fresh (preferably organic).
- Apple and lemon juice together, diluted.
- Fresh fruits and vegetables, raw and cooked.
- Fruit and vegetable juices—fruit in the morning, vegetables in the afternoon.
- Juices plus spirulina, algae, or other green chlorophyll powders.
- Whole grains, cooked squashes, and other vegetables (a lighter detox).
- Mixture of the above plans, with garlic as a prime detoxifier.
- Basic low-toxicity diet, with additional herbal program.
- Colon detox with fiber (psyllium, pectin, etc.) along with enemas or colonics.
- Prepare and plan a new autumn diet, enhancing positive dietary habits.

~ MID-AUTUMN ~

Take a 3-day cleanse with juices or in-season produce in late October to early November.

~ WINTER ~

A lighter diet, eaten for a week or two in preparation for the holidays (or as detox from them) can be done between December 10 and January 5:

- Avoid toxins and treats; eat a very basic wholesome diet.
- One week of brown rice, cooked vegetables, miso broth, and seaweed. Ginger and cayenne pepper can be used in soups.
- Saunas or steams and massage—you deserve it!
- Hang on until spring!

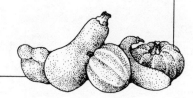

WHERE Can We Detoxify?

During basic, simple detoxification programs, most of us can maintain our normal daily routine. In fact, energy, performance, and health often improve. For some, the detox process may produce headaches, fatigue, irritability, mucous congestions, or aches and pains for the first few days. Any of the symptoms of toxicity may appear, however usually they don't. Symptoms that have been experienced previously may reoccur transiently during detoxification; sometimes it is hard to know whether or not to treat them. Since my approach to medicine is to allow the body to heal itself, I try to support the natural healing process whenever possible unless the person is very uncomfortable or the practitioner is concerned.

It is wise to begin new programs, diets, or lifestyle changes with a few days at home. In time, experience will show what works best. Most of us can maintain a regular work schedule during a cleanse or detox program (and we may even be more productive). However, it might be easier to begin a program on a Friday, as the first few days are usually the hardest. Some of us may be more sensitive during cleansing to the stress of our work environment or to chemical exposures. Also, co-workers or family members may provide temptations or challenge our decisions. Having supportive guides or co-cleansers can be a great comfort and source of positive reinforcement when our inner resolve begins to fade. At the end of the first or second day, usually around dinnertime, symptoms like headache and fatigue may begin to appear, and it is good to be able to rest and spend time in familiar, undemanding surroundings. By the third day, we usually feel pretty stable and ready for work.

Still, many people like to start new programs on a Monday, knowing that they will do fine, using willpower and visualization to see themselves through. People often feel better than ever and are able to accomplish tasks and meet challenges more easily than usual. In fact, experienced fasters may *utilize fasting* during busy work periods to improve their productivity. Preparing and planning, clearing doubts and fears, and keeping a daily journal are all useful during this vital process and are crucial to any successful undertaking.

WHY Detoxify?

We detoxify/cleanse for health, vitality, and rejuvenation—to clear symptoms, treat disease, and prevent future problems. A cleansing program is an ideal way to help us reevaluate our lives, make changes, or clear abuses and addictions. Withdrawal happens fairly rapidly, and as cravings are reduced we can begin a new life without the addictive habits or drugs.

I cleanse because it makes me feel more vital, creative, and open to emotional and spiritual energies. Many people detox/cleanse (or, more commonly, fast on water or juices) for spiritual renewal and to feel more alive, awake, and aware. Jesus Christ, Paramahansa Yogananda, Mahatma Ghandi, Dr. Martin Luther King, and many other spiritual and religious teachers have advocated fasting for spiritual and physical health.

Detoxification can be helpful for weight loss, although this is not its primary purpose, *I think cleansing is more important as an overall lifestyle and dietary transition.* However, just the simplification of our diet will have some detoxifying effects in our body. Anyone eating 4,000 calories daily of fatty, sweet foods in a poorly balanced diet, who begins to eat 2,000–2,500 calories daily of more wholesome foods will definitely experience detoxification, weight loss, and improved health simultaneously.

We also cleanse/detoxify to rest or heal our overloaded digestive organs and allow them to catch up on past work. At the same time, we are inspired to cleanse our external life as well, cleaning out rooms, sorting through the piles on our desks, clarifying our personal priorities, or revitalizing our wardrobes. Most often our energy is increased and becomes more steady, motivating us to change both internally and externally.

REASONS FOR CLEANSING		
Prevent disease	Clear skin	Productive
Reduce symptoms	Slow aging	Relaxed
Treat disease	Improve flexibility	Energetic
Cleanse body	Improve fertility	Conscious
Rest organs	Enhance the senses	Inwardly attuned
Purification	*To be more:*	Spiritual
Rejuvenation	Creative	Environmentally attuned
Weight loss	Motivated	Relationship focused

Hygiene Awareness

Proper hygiene inside and outside our body and personal environment is one of the four laws of good health, along with eating an alkaline-based diet of whole foods, exercising daily, and having proper rest, relaxation, and recreation. Although I believe that germs have a harder time causing problems in a healthy body, they do cause certain kinds of problems from mild colds and flus to life-threatening infections. Therefore, do what you can to protect yourself and do not share your germs too freely with others.

HEALTHY HYGIENE HINTS

1. Wash your hands several times daily—especially after eliminating, before handling food, after handling animals/pets, when you are sick with an upper respiratory problem (coughing, sneezing, or runny nose), or when you are in close physical contact with others. Also, clean up after a public encounter, such as hand-shaking, door-opening, or using public phones.

2. Bathe or shower at least once daily, more if you are sweaty or dirty, in a clean tub or shower; also, use environmentally-friendly hygiene products and cleansers.

3. Exercise and sweat regularly to help cleanse your skin and move the lymphatic fluids.

4. Keep your nails clean and cut, and clear out dirt and germs that may get under them with hydrogen peroxide or a nail brush.

5. Do not put used utensils or your hands into group food.

6. Blow your nose and rinse out your nose and sinuses when you are congested.

7. Follow safe sex guidelines, especially with a new partner.

8. Make sure your diet and activity level facilitate at least one to two good bowel movements a day and clean yourself properly afterwards.

9. Keep your kitchen and refrigerator clean; wash counters and cutting boards regularly. Don't let germs breed in your trash bins—wash them regularly as well.

10. Minimize your use of and exposure to chemicals at home and in the workplace. Don't replace germs and dirt with chemicals.

CHAPTER THREE

The Detox Diet and Other Diets for Detoxification

Before we approach the Detox Diet, I first want to give you a little preventive medicine—some guidelines to follow so that you don't *need* to detoxify. Instead, learn to eat and live in a way that creates and supports health, vitality, and longevity. The first step is to follow a nontoxic diet. If we do this regularly, we have less need for cleansing. If we have not been eating this way, we should detoxify first and then make these more permanent changes.

THE NONTOXIC DIET

- Eat organic foods whenever possible.

- Drink filtered water.

- Rotate foods, especially common allergens such as milk products, eggs, wheat, and yeast foods.

- Practice food combining.

- Eat a natural, seasonal cuisine.

- Include fruits, vegetables, whole grains, legumes, nuts, and seeds, and, for omnivarians, some low- or non-fat dairy products, fresh fish (not shellfish), and organic poultry.

- Cook in iron, stainless steel, glass, or porcelain cookware.

- Avoid or minimize red meats, cured meats, organ meats, refined foods, canned foods, sugar, salt, saturated fats, coffee, alcohol, and nicotine.

Another aspect of the nontoxic diet is avoiding drugs (over-the-counter, prescription, and recreational) and substituting natural remedies such as nutritional supplements, herbs, and homeopathic medicines, all of which have fewer side effects.[*] Other natural therapies, such as acupuncture, massage, osteopathic, and chiropractic care may help in treating certain problems so that we will not *need* drugs for them. Avoiding or minimizing exposure to chemicals at home and at work is also important. One way we can do this is by substituting natural cleansers, cosmetics, and clothing.

One of my favorite cleansing/detox programs is the Detox Diet. It is a simple eating program that I have used with many hundreds of people. I find it to be a great catalyst for healing, providing more energy, fewer debilitating symptoms, and the inspiration necessary for making permanent changes in diet and lifestyle habits.

When I did my first 3-week Detox Diet, I learned to chew my food thoroughly for the first time in my life. I felt more nourished on less food and I experienced less bloating, gas, and fullness within several hours of eating. My weight dropped five pounds per week and I felt clearer, more energized, and less congested.

Over the last five years, I have prescribed this Detox Diet for those with obvious congestion-toxicity concerns, such as people with high blood pressure who are also overweight and stressed, those with arthritis and joint pains, allergies, or recurrent sinus problems, or those with back pains or lymphatic congestion. Most people experience similar results—a couple of days of transition with occasional fatigue, irritability, hunger, or increased congestion. Usually by the third day they start to feel cleaner, clearer, lighter, stronger, and more present in their body, aware of the way it responds to food and liquid intake. Their symptoms of congestion and pain diminish and even disappear. It is very gratifying for them and myself and often represents a long-term change, and it certainly makes my job more enjoyable and rewarding.

[*] See p. 61 for advice on transitioning from pharmaceutical to natural therapies.

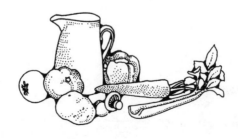

THE DETOX DIET DAILY MENU PLAN

Upon rising:

Two glasses of water (filtered or spring), one glass with half a lemon squeezed into it.

Breakfast:

One piece of fresh fruit (at room temperature), such as an apple, pear, banana, a citrus fruit, or some grapes. Chew well, mixing each bite with saliva.

Fifteen to thirty minutes later: One bowl of cooked whole grains—specifically millet, brown rice, amaranth, quinoa, or buckwheat.

For flavoring, use two tablespoons of fruit juice for sweetness, or use the Better Butter mentioned below with a little salt or tamari for a savory taste.

Lunch:

(Noon-1 PM) One to two medium bowls of steamed vegetables; use a variety, including roots, stems, and greens. For example, potatoes or yams, green beans, broccoli or cauliflower, carrots or beets, asparagus, kale, chard, and cabbage. Be sure to *chew well!*

Dinner:

(5-6 PM) Same as lunch.

Make Better Butter by mixing a quarter-cup of cold-pressed canola oil into a soft (room temperature) quarter-pound of butter; then place in dish and refrigerate. Use about one teaspoon per meal or a maximum of 3 teaspoons daily.

Special drinks:

(11 AM and 3 PM)

One to two cups veggie water, saved from the steamed vegetables. Add a little sea salt or kelp and drink slowly, mixing each mouthful with saliva.

Before retiring:

Consume no additional foods after dinner. Drink only water and herbal teas, such as peppermint, chamomile, pau d'arco, or blends.

Seasonal Vegetable Suggestions

Try steaming basic combinations that include some root vegetables, tubers, stems, leafy greens, and vegetables fruits (from flowering vines that give such veggies as zucchini, green beans, and peppers).

~ SPRING ~

Asparagus, baby carrots, spring garlic, red chard, beets, leeks, broccoli.
Wild greens such as mustard, sorrel or collard, with a steamed artichoke.

~ SUMMER ~

Zucchini, new potatoes, green beans, carrots, onion.
Beets and beet greens, yellow squash, bell pepper, eggplant.

~ AUTUMN ~

Broccoli, cabbage, potato, celery, spinach.
Cauliflower, onion, carrots, chard, sugar peas.

~ WINTER~

Broccoli, cabbage, potato, kale, spinach, chard.
Butternut squash, onion, cauliflower, collard greens, Jerusalem artichoke.

To season, add a little bit of sea salt, vegetable salt, or a good garlic salt without additives, or cayenne for warmth. Better Butter (see recipe, p. 35) is a must for the Alkaline-Detoxification Menu Plan as it prevents deficiencies of essential fatty acids. The mixture of butter and cold-pressed canola oil provides all the fatty acids to nourish and support the tissues.

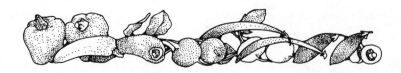

The effects of dietary detoxification vary. Even mild changes from our current eating plan will produce some responses, while more dramatic dietary shifts can produce a profound cleansing. Shifting from the most congesting foods to the least—eating more fruits, vegetables, grains, nuts, and legumes and less baked goods, sweets, refined foods, fried foods, and fatty foods—will help most of us detoxify somewhat and bring us into better balance overall.

Maintaining the same diet but adding certain supplements such as fiber, vitamin C, other antioxidants, chlorophyll, and glutathione (mainly as amino acid L-cysteine) can also stimulate detoxification. Herbs such as garlic, red clover, echinacea, or cayenne may also induce some detoxification as can saunas, sweats, and niacin therapy. (See Chapter Four for more discussion of supplements.) Simply increasing liquid intake and decreasing fats and refined flour products will improve elimination and lessen toxin buildup. Increased consumption of filtered water, herb teas, fruits, and vegetables while reducing fats (especially fried foods, red meat, and milk products) will also help detoxification. A vegetarian diet may also be a healthful step for those with some congestive problems. Meats, milk products, breads, and baked goods (especially refined sugar and carbohydrate products) increase body acidity and lead to more mucus production as the body attempts to balance its chemistry. The more alkaline vegetarian foods enhance cleansing. *The right balance of acid and alkaline foods for each of us is, of course, the key.**

Acid and Alkaline—A Key to Health and Longevity

The acid-alkaline state is crucial to what scientists call the biological **terrain** of the body, or the state of the body's tissues and functions. I believe that it is this terrain that affects whether or not we are healthy. Parasitic, fungal, and other infections are secondary to imbalances of the terrain; diet, stress levels, and other aspects of lifestyle can profoundly influence it. Since animal products, refined foods (sugars and flours), nuts, and seeds are more acidic in their chemical makeup, they create acid residues when metabolized in the body. They contain higher amounts of the minerals **phosphorus, sulfur, chlorine,** and **iodine,** while the more alkaline-generating foods contain higher levels of **calcium, magnesium, potassium,** and **sodium.** These include most high water-content fruits and vegetables, as well as some grains and almonds.

---

* See chapters 10 and 12 of *Staying Healthy with Nutrition* for more information on acid and alkaline.

Over time, the consumption of an animal-product based diet creates an acidic state of the tissues, with chronic congestions, inflammation, toxicity, and degeneration. The end-point of this process is the many painful and terminal diseases people experience as they age.

Over the years I have measured and had patients follow their own pH, or acid, levels—assessing their blood, urine, and saliva, and then monitoring any changes, especially in urine and saliva—to chart their course of healing. There is clearly a strong correlation between body fluid pH and the level of health or disease of the individual. If our tissues accumulate more acid, the kidneys attempt to release acid and withhold bicarbonate, which makes the blood more alkaline.

Acid states appear in people with acute and chronic inflammatory and pain syndromes, congestive disorders that include recurrent infections and allergies, and the degenerative diseases such as cancer, cardiovascular problems, and diabetes. Once these chronic degenerative diseases have set in, they are more difficult to treat or correct. When I have been able to assess and rebalance an individual's biochemistry, I have seen the lessening of symptoms, the halt of disease progression, and even the reversal of some conditions—and I have experienced this with thousands of patients.

And now the **Detox Diet**, or, more clearly, the **Alkaline Detoxification Diet**—the smoothest, long-range transitional and healing program available. It is the great biochemical balancer for the person consuming the typical Western diet, a diet that I have worked diligently to try to change both personally and professionally.

A more rigorous detox diet is one made up exclusively of fresh fruits, fresh vegetables (either raw or cooked), and whole grains (both cooked and sprouted). No breads or baked goods, animal foods or dairy products, alcohol or nuts are used. This diet keeps fiber and water intake up and hence helps colon detoxification. Most people can handle this quite easily and make the shift from their regular diet with only a few days transition. Others prefer a brown rice fast (a more macrobiotic approach) for a week or two, eating three to four bowls of rice daily along with liquids such as green or herbal teas.

An even deeper level of detoxification involves a diet consisting solely of fruits and vegetables—all cleansing foods. The green vegetables, especially the chlorophyllic and high-nutrient leafy greens, support purification of the gastrointestinal tract.

A raw foods diet is fulfilling for many people, yielding high energy and quality nutrition. It utilizes sprouted greens from seeds and grains such as wheat, buckwheat, sunflower, alfalfa, and clover; sprouted beans such as mung or garbanzo; soaked or sprouted raw nuts; and fresh fruits and vegetables. Cooked food is not allowed with this diet, as eating foods raw maintains the highest concentrations of vitamins, minerals, and important enzymes. Many people feel that this is the best diet, and I think it can be supportive over quite some time if it is properly balanced. Detox-healing diets are also available specifically for problems such as yeast overgrowth or food allergies.

The liquid cleanses or fasts move beyond the alkaline detoxification and fruit-and-vegetable diets. Juices, vegetable broths, and teas can be used to purify our body during fasting. Miso soup, made from a paste of fermented soybean, also provides many nutrients and supports colon function by aiding the intestinal bacteria. Spirulina (an algae powder) or blue-green fresh water algae can also be helpful to fasters who experience fatigue by providing amino acids for protein building (add to juices for best flavor).

Water fasting is more intense than fasting with juices, and often results in more sickness and less energy. Paavo Airola, one of the pioneers of fasting in America, states in *How to Get Well* that, "systematic undereating and periodic fasting are the two most important health and longevity factors." Consuming fresh, diluted juices from various fruits and vegetables can be a safe and helpful approach for many conditions. Further, specific juice regimes may be used beneficially by people for whom water fasts are contraindicated. Juices help to eliminate wastes and dead cells while building new tissue with the easily accessible nutrients.

The key to proper treatment is to individualize your program. I look at the patient's general health, physiological balance, energy level, and current lifestyle in order to set up the right program. If you are unsure, start with the basic diet and gradually intensify toward juice fasting and see how you feel. Take a couple of days for each step, and, if you feel fine, move to the next level as described here:

Levels of Dietary Detoxification

- Basic diet
- Reduce toxins daily ingesting fewer congesting foods and more nourishing ones (see chart on page 26); for example, decrease drugs, sugar, fried foods, meats, dairy, etc. Take one to seven days.
- Fruits, vegetables, whole grains, nuts, seeds, and legumes
- Raw foods
- Fruits and vegetables
- Fruit and vegetable juices
- Specific juice diets, Master Cleanser, apple, carrot, and greens, etc. (See Chapter 10: Fasting and Juice Cleansing.)
- Water

When I set up an initial detox/cleansing program, I evaluate each individual with a health history, physical exam, biochemical tests, dietary analysis, and mineral level evaluation. By interpreting the patient's current symptoms and disease as a result of their diet, lifestyle, and genetic patterns, and by then considering their current health goals, we can create a plan together. As is true with any healing process, the plan must be reevaluated and fine-tuned to the individual to make it work optimally over time.

If the patient is deficient in nutrients and/or energy, she may need a higher-protein, higher-nutrient rebuilding diet—greater nourishment rather than a cleanse to improve her health. Fatigue, mineral deficiencies, and low organ functions may call for this more supportive, nourishing diet. However, even in these circumstances, short three-day cleanses can help eliminate old debris and prepare the body to build with healthier blocks.

Our individual detox programs do change, as our needs often vary with time. For instance, my own personal program has changed in intensity over the decades. Initially, fasts were very powerful, transformative, and healing for me. Now I feel much cleaner most of the time and I usually notice less effect from a fast. If I do get congested with different foods, travel, or when under stress, a few days of juices or light eating will make a big difference. I ate a low-protein, high-complex-carbohydrate vegetarian diet for a number of years; now my mild detox consists of more strengthening protein-vegetable meals. Fresh fish with lots of vegetables satisfies and energizes me more now than it did in the past.[*] My previous higher-starch diet led me to overeat in order to feel nourished. This new diet has let me reduce calories and weight while feeling stronger and healthier. And this too, I am sure, will change over time.

---

[*] The oceans are polluted like everything else. Deep sea fish such as sole, tuna, and halibut seem to be the cleanest choices.

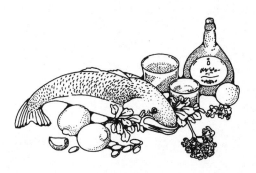

CHAPTER FOUR

Supplements for Detoxification

◆

Colon cleansing is one of the most important steps in detoxification. The large intestine releases many toxins, and sluggish functioning of this organ can rapidly produce general toxicity. During any detox program, most people will incorporate some colon cleansing. Helpful products include herbal or pharmaceutical laxatives, fiber, and colon detox supplements such as psyllium seed husks alone or mixed with other agents (such as aloe vera powder, betonite clay, and acidophilus culture). Enemas using water, herbs, or even diluted coffee (the latter of which stimulates liver cleansing) may also be used. A series of colonic water irrigations (best performed by a trained professional with filtered water and sterile, disposable equipment) can be the focal point of a detox program accompanied by a cleansing diet and fiber supplements.* Whatever the method, keeping the bowels moving is key to feeling well during detoxification.

Regular exercise is also very important as it stimulates sweating and encourages elimination through the skin. Exercise also improves our general metabolism and helps overall with detoxification. For this reason, regular aerobic exercise is key to maintaining a nontoxic body, especially when we indulge in various substances such as sugar or alcohol. Since exercise releases toxins in the body, it is important to incorporate adequate fluids, antioxidants, vitamins, and minerals.

Regular bathing cleanses the skin of toxins that have been released and opens the pores for further elimination, and are particularly beneficial during detoxification. Saunas and sweats are commonly used to enhance skin elimination. Dry brushing the skin with an appropriate skin brush before bathing is also suggested to invigorate the skin and cleanse away old cells. Massage therapy (especially lymphatic or deep massage) stimulates elimination and body functions and promotes relaxation. Clearing generalized tensions also makes for a more complete detoxification.

---

* There are also entire programs for colon detoxification available, such as Dr. Robert Gray's Colon Cleansing program (which includes a book and special supplements) found mainly in health food stores. For a complete body and colon cleansing program, I really like Nature's Pure Body Program available through their toll-free number (800) 952-7873.

Resting, relaxation, and recharging are also important to this rejuvenation process. During the detox process, we may need more rest, quiet time, and sleep, although more commonly we have more energy and function better on less sleep than before. Relaxation exercises help our body rebalance itself as our mind and attitudes stop interfering with our natural homeostasis. The practice of yoga combines quiet yet powerful exercises with breath awareness and regulation, allowing increased flexibility and relaxation.

Certain supplements are appropriate for some detoxification programs. However, general supplementation may be less important in this detox program than with the specific detox plans for alcohol, caffeine, and nicotine when more nutrients can ease withdrawal symptoms. For straight juice cleansing or water fasts, I usually do not recommend very many supplements; however, I may suggest a couple of nutrients or herbs to stimulate the detoxification process. Examples include potassium, extra fiber with olive oil to clear toxins from the colon, sodium alginate from seaweeds to bind heavy metals, and apple cider vinegar in water (1 tablespoon vinegar in 8 ounces hot water) to help reduce mucus. I have used blue-green algae, chlorella, and spirulina before, as I and other fasters often feel better and more energetic when we use these nutrient-rich foods. For people who begin with transition diets, I usually suggest a specialized nutrient program to help neutralize toxins and support elimination. With weight loss (for detoxers who are overweight), toxins stored in the fat will need to be mobilized and cleared—more water, fiber, and antioxidant nutrients can help handle this.

The supplement program used for general detoxification (with additional support to reduce nutrient deficiency during detox) is outlined in the table at the end of this chapter. It includes a low-dosage multiple vitamin/mineral supplement to fulfill the basic nutritional requirements during the transitional diet. The B vitamins, particularly niacin, are also important, as are minerals such as zinc, calcium, magnesium, and potassium. The antioxidant nutrients include beta-carotene, vitamin A, zinc, vitamin E, selenium, and especially vitamin C. Some authorities believe that higher amounts of vitamin A (10,000 IU), Beta-Carotene (25,000-50,000 IU), vitamin C (8–12 g), and vitamin E (1,000–1,200 IU) are helpful during detoxification to neutralize the free radicals.

The liver is our most important detoxification organ. Because of this, liver-supportive nutrients and liver glandulars are often suggested during general detoxification. The liver needs water and glycogen (stored glucose) as glucuronic acid for many of its detoxifying functions—a higher starch or carbohydrate diet, if tolerated, with lower levels of protein and fats can supply this. The B vitamins, especially B_3 and B_6, vitamins A and C, zinc, calcium, vitamin E and selenium, and L-cysteine are all also needed to support liver detoxification. Milk thistle herb (often sold as silymarin or *Silybum marianum)* has also been shown to aid liver detoxification and repair.

Several amino acids improve or support detoxification, particularly cysteine and methionine, which contain sulfur. L-cysteine supplies sulfhydryl groups which help prevent oxidation and bind heavy metals such as mercury; vitamin C and selenium aid this process. Cysteine is the precursor to glutathione—our most important detoxifier—which counters many chemicals and carcinogens. Glutathione is synthesized to form detoxification enzymes *glutathione peroxidase* and *reductase*, which work to prevent peroxidation of lipids and to decrease toxins such as smoke, radiation, auto exhaust, chemicals, drugs, and other carcinogens.

Glycine is a secondary helper. An amino acid that supports glutathione synthesis, glycine decreases the toxicity of substances such as phenols or benzoic acid (a food preservative). Glutamine is also important in helping to heal the GI tract as well as reduce cravings for sugar and alcohol, should they occur. Other amino acids that may have mild detoxifying effects are methionine, tyrosine, and taurine.[*]

As mentioned earlier, fiber also supports detoxification. Psyllium seed husks (often combined with other detox nutrients, such as pectin, aloe vera, alginates, and/or colon herbs) help cleanse mucus along the small intestine, create bulk in the colon, and pull toxins from the gastrointestinal tract. When fiber is combined with one or two tablespoons of olive oil, it helps bind toxins and reduce the absorption of fats and some basic minerals. Psyllium husks also reduce absorption of the olive oil itself, which is important in reducing calories and binding any fat-soluble chemicals that may have been released. In *Vitamin Power*, Stephanie Rick and Rita Aero suggest taking 1-2 teaspoons each of psyllium and bran several times daily (with meals and at bedtime) along with one teaspoon of olive oil to help detoxify the colon. Acidophilus bacteria in the colon neutralizes some toxins, reduces the metabolism of other microbes, and lessens colon toxicity. Supplemental acidophilus is often added to a detox program.

---

[*] For more information on amino acid metabolism and uses, I suggest a book by Dr. Eric R. Braverman and the late Dr. Carl C. Pfieffer entitled *The Healing Nutrients Within: Facts, Findings and New Research on Amino Acids* (New Canaan, CT: Keats Publishing, Inc.) , or see Chapter 3 in *Staying Healthy with Nutrition*

Water

Remember, water is crucial to any type of detox program for diluting and eliminating toxin accumulations. It is probably our most important detoxifier as it helps us clean through our skin and kidneys, and improves our sweating with exercise. Eight to ten glasses a day (depending on body size and activity level) of clean, filtered water are suggested. Some authorities suggest distilled water for use during detox programs, as its lack of minerals draws other particles (nutrients and toxins) to it. I think it throws off our biochemical/electrical balance, and hence prefer regular, purified water. I recommend two or three glasses of water 30 to 60 minutes before each meal (and at night) to help flush toxins during our body's natural elimination time.

Niacin-Sauna Therapy

A special detoxification process has been developed to help in the release of chemicals, pesticides, and pharmaceutical drugs. Used in some clinics, this program includes several weeks of a high-fluid and juice diet, exercise, and a high intake of niacin (vitamin B_3) with sauna therapy.[*] The extended saunas may last several hours, with breaks to drink fluids. Niacin is a vasostimulator and vasodilator, aiding circulation. The idea is to cleanse hidden chemicals from fat through juice cleansing, weight loss, niacin therapy, exercise, and sweats.

The niacin-sauna program has therapeutic possibilities as an intense, medically-supervised detoxification process; however, it is still experimental and does entail risks. Preliminary results are good—especially for people with symptoms caused by exposure to pesticides such as Agent Orange—yet there are some drawbacks. The program is costly and time-consuming. This extreme detox can also cause nutrient deficiencies which can take months to replenish. Proper nutrient restoration must be ensured, both during and after this therapy. This program does help detoxification from many chemicals and drugs (especially the recreational types) and from daily abuses of alcohol and nicotine. Many of us can do a modified version of this therapy on our own with sauna, a few days of juice cleansing, regular exercise, and supplemental niacin (beginning at 100–200 mg and moving up to 2–3 grams daily). Be sure to replenish fluids and minerals. If you have any pre-existing medical problems, weakness, or fatigue, I suggest seeing a physician first.

[*] This therapy is available now in the new Healthcare for the 21st Century Clinic in Manhattan, directed by Adrienne Buffaloe, M.D., (see page 127).

Herbs

Many herbs support or even instigate detoxification, and I believe that this is the real strength of herbal medicine. Hundreds of herbal possibilities exist for blood cleansing, tissue cleaning, or strengthening the function of specific organs. The following are some of the more important ones.

CLEANSING HERBS

Garlic—blood cleanser, lowers blood fats, natural antibiotic

Red clover blossoms—blood cleanser, good during convalescence and healing

Echinacea—lymph cleanser, improves lymphocyte and phagocyte actions, immunity supporter, antimicrobial

Dandelion root—liver and blood cleanser, diuretic, filters toxins, a tonic

Chaparral—strong blood cleanser, with possibilities for use in cancer therapy

Cayenne pepper—blood and tissue purifier, increases fluid elimination and sweat, a natural stimulant

Cascara sagrada—a colon cleanser and tonic

Ginger root—stimulates circulation and sweating, relieves congestion

Licorice root—the "great detoxifier," biochemical balancer, mild laxative

Yellow dock root—skin, blood, and liver cleanser, contains vitamin C and iron

Burdock root—skin and blood cleanser, diuretic and diaphoretic, improves liver function, antibacterial and antifungal properties

Sarsaparilla root—blood and lymph cleanser, contains saponins, which reduce microbes and toxins

Prickly ash bark—good for nerves and joints, anti-infectious

Oregon grape root—skin and colon cleanser, blood purifier, liver stimulant

Parsley leaf—diuretic, flushes kidneys

Goldenseal root—blood, liver, kidney, and skin cleanser, stimulates detoxification

---

A General Classification of Herbs Useful in Detoxification*

Blood Cleansers
Echinacea
Red clover
Dandelion
Burdock
Yellow dock
Oregon grape root

Laxatives/Colon Cleansers
Cascara sagrada
Buckthorn
Dandelion
Yellow dock
Rhubarb root
Senna leaf
Licorice

Diuretics
Parsley
Yarrow
Cleavers
Horsetail
Corn silk
Uva ursi
Juniper berries

Skin Cleansers (Diaphoretics)
Burdock
Oregon grape
Yellow dock
Goldenseal
Boneset
Elder flowers
Peppermint
Cayenne pepper
Ginger root

Antibiotics
Garlic
Myrrh
Prickly ash
Wormwood
Echinacea
Propolis
Clove
Eucalyptus

Anticatarrhals**
Echinacea
Boneset
Goldenseal
Sage
Hyssop
Garlic
Yarrow

* Not usually used with fasting or juice cleansing, but as supplements to dietary detoxification—using herbs alone may be the most productive in some detoxification programs. Consult a naturopathically oriented doctor.
** Anticatarrhals help eliminate mucus.

Sample Detox Formula

Echinacea   **Cayenne pepper**   **Parsley leaf**
Goldenseal root   **Garlic**   **Licorice root**
Yellow dock root

Obtain powders (or ground herbs) in equal amounts for all of the above except cayenne, for which you should get half. Mix and put into 00 capsules. Take two capsules two or three times daily between meals.

General Detoxification Nutrient Program

The following supplements tie together many aspects of detoxification. Individual circumstances should be taken into account when determining which supplements to use. The program can be carried out for varying lengths of time, ranging from one week to one or two months. Programs for specific detox situations are described in the following chapters. Remember to incorporate all levels of detoxification and listen to your body as it gives its unique, individual response to these healing agents and processes.

GENERAL DETOXIFICATION NUTRIENT PROGRAM—DAILY AMOUNTS

Water	2 1/2–3 qt	Biotin	200 mcg
Fiber	20–40 g	Vitamin C	1–4 g
Vitamin A	5,000-7,500 IU	Bioflavonoids	250–500 mg
Beta-carotene	15,000-30,000 IU	Calcium	600–850 mg
Vitamin D	200-400 IU	Chromium	200 mcg
Vitamin E	400–1,000 IU	Copper	2 mg
Vitamin K	200 mcg	Iodine	150 mcg
Thiamine (B$_1$)	10–25 mg	Magnesium	300–500 mg
Riboflavin (B$_2$)	10–25 mg	Manganese	5–10 mg
Niacinamide (B$_3$)	50 mg	Molybdenum	300 mcg
Niacin (B$_3$)	50–2,000 mg*	Potassium	300–500 mg
Pantothenic acid (B$_5$)	250-500 mg	Selenium	300 mcg
Pyridoxine (B$_6$)	10–25 mg	Silicon	100 mg
Cobalamin (B$_{12}$)	50–100 mcg	Vanadium	300 mcg
Folic acid	400–800 mcg	Zinc	30 mg

OPTIONAL

L-amino acids (general blend)	500–1,000 mg	Olive oil	3–6 teaspoons
L-cysteine	250–500 mg	Liquid chlorophyll	2–4 teaspoons
DL-methionine	250–500 mg	Apple cider vinegar	1–2 Tablespoons
L-glycine	250–500 mg		
L-glutamine	500-1,000 mg		
Psyllium seed	2-4 teaspoons or 8-12 caps		
Flaxseed oil	1–2 teaspoons or 2-4 caps		
Acidophilus culture	more than 2 billion organisms/day		
Detox formula herbs:	4–6 capsules		
echinacea, yellow dock, goldenseal, garlic, parsley, licorice, cayenne pepper			

*May be used for special detox programs; see previous discussion.

CHAPTER FIVE

Sugar Detoxification

◆

For most of us, sugar is a symbol of love and nurturance because as infants, our first food is lactose, or milk sugar. Overconsumption and daily use of sugar is the first compulsive habit for most everyone with addictions later in life. Simple sugar, or glucose, is what our body, our cells, and brain use as fuel for energy. Some glucose is stored in our liver and muscle tissues as glycogen for future use; excess sugar is stored as fat for use during periods of low-calorie intake or starvation.

Our problem with sweets comes from the frequency with which we eat them, and the quantity of sugar we consume. The type of sugar we eat is also a contributing factor. Refined sugar or sucrose (a disaccharide made up of two sugars—glucose and fructose) is usually extracted from sugar cane or sugar beets, initially whole foods. However, most all of the nutrients are removed and retained only in the discarded extract called molasses. When the manufacturing process is complete, the result is pure sugar, a refined crystal that contains four calories per gram and essentially no nutrients.

Sugar and sweeteners have so pervaded our food manufacturing and restaurant industries that it is almost impossible to find prepackaged products which are unsweetened. Most frequently used are both refined, high-calorie, non-nutrient sucrose, and the corn syrup derivatives, or one of the more recent and common "invisible sweeteners." Consequently, the only way to avoid sweeteners is to avoid packaged products whenever possible. Fruits contain natural fructose, in balance with other nutrients; honey and maple syrup are more highly concentrated natural sugars and are appropriate for most of us in moderation.

Traditional Chinese Medicine views the desire for sugar, or the sweet flavor, as a craving for the mother (yin) energy, a craving that represents a need for comfort or security. A desire for spicy or salty flavored foods might represent looking for the father (yang) energy or power and direction. In Western cultures, we have turned sugar into a reward system (a tangible symbol of material nurturing) to the degree that many of us have been conditioned to need some sweet treat to feel complete or satisfied. We continue these patterns with our children, unconsciously showing our affection for them by giving them sugary foods. Holidays and special occasions are centered around sugar—birthday cakes and ice cream, Halloween candy, chocolate Easter eggs, Thanksgiving pie, Christmas cookies, Valentine chocolates—the list is endless. We even reward our children for good behavior by giving them treats. Sweet talk is embedded in our language—sweetie, sweetie pie, sweetheart, honey, honey pie, sugar, sugar baby, candy, sweet cakes, baby cakes, honey bun, sugar plum. The message is loud and clear: sweetness=love.

Sugar and Health

Many nutritional authorities feel that the high use of sugar in our diet is a significant underlying cause of disease. Too much sweetener in any form can have a negative effect on our health; this includes not only refined sugar, but also corn syrup, honey and fruit juices, and treats such as sodas, cakes, and candies. Because sugary foods satisfy our hunger, they often replace more nutritious foods and weaken our tissue's health and disease resistance.

PROBLEMS ASSOCIATED WITH SUGAR INTAKE*

Tooth Decay

Obesity and its increased risk of **Diabetes, Cancer,** and other diseases

Nutritional Deficiency—including anemia, protein and mineral deficiencies

Hypoglycemia and Carbohydrate imbalance

Chronic Dyspepsia and digestive problems

Immune Dysfunction and problems such as recurrent infections

Menstrual Irregularities & Premenstrual Symptoms (PMS)

Yeast Overgrowth and its many subsequent problems, including craving sweets and carbohydrates

Hyperactivity and difficulty concentrating

Alcoholism—a potential link as it is associated with hypoglycemia and abnormal carbohydrate metabolism

Mood swings, anxiety, depression

Heart Disease

There is much evidence that eating too many sweets eventually causes disease. If these conditions occur in either your personal or family history, it is important to seriously consider a dietary change for your health's sake.

Sugar can also compromise our body's ability to fight illness. In 1976, Emanuel Cheraskin, MD. and others showed that a single intake of sugar can lower the bacteria-fighting capabilities of white blood cells (phagocytic activity) in the blood of test subjects for up to five hours. In a number of other studies, researchers found a positive correlation between sugar overconsumption and eight forms of cancer—colon, rectum, breast, ovary, prostate, kidney, nervous system, and pancreas. In some cases, the risk was more than doubled by consuming sugar on a regular basis.

A connection between high sugar intake and coronary artery disease was discovered in 1964. Research in 1993 revealed that alteration in carbohydrate metabolism is a significant risk factor for the development of cardiovascular disease. This is especially true for women who take birth control pills or hormones.

Impaired glucose tolerance is also described as one of the strongest predictors of adult-onset (noninsulin-dependent) diabetes. With insulin-dependent diabetes, positive actions to manage sugar and starch intake can help protect against associated secondary problems, such as neuropathy and blindness.

Digestive problems and chronic indigestion can result from excessive intake of sweets. *Candida albicans* and other microorganisms love sweet, simple, sugary foods. A sweet diet encourages greater infestation of bacteria, yeasts, and parasites, and will support their growth. Microbe infestation can also weaken our immunity. Additionally, the presence of candida and other unfriendly organisms in our gut or other organ systems increases our craving for sweets, creating and perpetuating a negative cycle.

Frequent cravings for sweets can also be related to hypoglycemia (low blood sugar). Chronic low blood sugar can be the result of poor adrenal and pancreas function. However, we all get low blood sugar from time to time, when we skip a meal or work extra hard. If our blood sugar is low, a candy bar, a piece of cake, or an alcoholic beverage furnishes a quick "pick me up," reducing the symptoms of shakiness, fatigue, or anxiety. However, this relief is only short term. Sugar is absorbed so rapidly into the blood that the pancreas over-reacts to balance the glucose level. This can cause a rapid drop in blood sugar, which may result in mood swings with depression or anger. Orthomolecular medicine has suggested that some alcoholism may result from such hypoglycemic mood swings. In such cases, continuing to drink keeps the blood sugar up and the anxiety level down, but with negative long-term effects.

Sugar cravings are experienced commonly by women premenstrually; and chocolate is a common first choice. In Oriental medicine, the regular use or overuse of sugar is thought to lead to menstrual irregularities and premenstrual problems.

Sugar excess may also cause our bodies to age more rapidly. In 1993, geriatric researchers found that high calorie intake is a significant dietary factor responsible for aging. Empty calories from sweeteners and sweet foods may give us quick energy, but they also increase our energy utilization which stresses and ages our bodies more rapidly.

Our teeth are also subject to the destructive effects of sugar. When refined sugar was introduced into the diets of native peoples such as the Eskimos, New Zealand Maoris, and Australian aborigines, the number of dental cavities increased dramatically. In Europe and Japan, when sugar was rationed during World War II, the rate of cavities fell significantly. Research consistently shows that sugar and sticky starches destroy dental enamel and cause plaque and decay. Sweetened beverages are also linked to increased cavities. A major U.S. survey found that the use of soft drinks or sweet juices three or more times per day between meals doubled the chances of developing cavities.

Sugar and Its Effects on Children

Life-time dietary habits are formed in infancy, so limiting the intake of sweets is of major importance. Blood sugar during infancy is less stable than later in childhood; thus babies are more susceptible to foods which rapidly raise and lower blood sugar. In fact, infant failure-to-thrive syndrome has been correlated with impaired carbohydrate metabolism, and specifically sucrose malabsorption. Some babies and young children develop chronic colic, cramping, and diarrhea from eating sugar, and this has been reported in the medical literature for more than 20 years

Learning problems, exaggerated hyperactivity, and moodiness in children have all been linked to a high-sugar diet. Psychologists have observed decreased performance and increased inappropriate behavior following sugar intake. For certain children with attention deficit disorder (ADD), these effects can be more extreme. Not surprisingly, researchers found that decreasing sugar decreased socially inappropriate behavior.

The long-term effects of a sweet diet may actually be more severe than the immediate concerns. The habits we establish when we are young set the stage for lifetime patterns. A diet of empty calories may be a factor in frequent infections and failure to thrive. Extensive childhood dental cavities may result in teeth damaged beyond repair as an adult. Hypoglycemia in youth may result in recurring depression or alcoholism later in life. Chronic candida (yeast) infections, resulting from the frequent intake of sweets and the use of antibiotics, may set the stage for a lifetime of digestive and energy problems. Overweight children may become overweight adults, with the attendant increased risks for diabetes, cancer, and heart disease.

Decreasing the Sugar in Our Diet

Our intake of sweets is increasing, especially with the use of hidden sweeteners. A quick look at the yearly statistics gives the impression that we are eating fewer sweets, because our sugar consumption has dropped from about 100 pounds a person to 64. Sounds good. However, our yearly intake of corn sweeteners has gone from about 20 pounds a person to more than 80. Our total intake of sweeteners is now about 150 pounds a year per person—almost a half pound of sweets per day.

Reducing sweeteners in our diet is a very real, positive step each of us can take. It requires an effort, but reducing our dietary load of sugar and sweeteners is of key importance for our health and our children's health.

SUGAR SUBSTANCES ADDED TO FOODS

Sucrose	Fructose	Dextrose
Honey	Malt syrup	Maple sugar
Corn syrup	High-fructose corn syrup	Artificial Sweeteners

AVOID SUGAR FOODS AND SNACKS

white sugar	candy	cake
soda pop	artificial juices	sweetened drinks
pies	puddings	cookies
ice cream	doughnuts	breakfast cereals
jello	corn syrup	liqueurs
jams & jellies	chewing gum	mixed drinks

AVOID HIDDEN SUGAR IN FOODS

baking mixes	breads	crackers
ketchup	relish	tartar sauce
salad dressings	cheese dips	soups
pickles	peanut butter	frankfurters
luncheon meats	prepared seafood	sausage
canned fruits	frozen vegetables	sweetened yogurt

Sugar Detox

Although sugar addiction is common, sugar withdrawal is usually physically mild, with periodic strong cravings. For those who are more sensitive to refined sugar or sweeteners, or who consume it in large amounts, genuine symptoms of abuse and withdrawal may occur. Some of these symptoms include fatigue, anxiety and irritability, depression and detachment, rapid heart rate and palpitations, and poor sleep. Most symptoms, if they do occur, last only a few days.

We can decide to cut down on or eliminate sugar quite easily by simply avoiding many of the sweet foods. There are plenty of nutritious nibbles to replace sugary snacks or treats—see below for suggestions. We should clear our cupboards of unhealthy sweetened foods. Once sugar has been removed from the diet, it is still possible to use it once in awhile, as it is not as readdicting as many stronger drugs. Most people who have kicked the sugar habit find that they no longer tolerate sugar very well.

GOOD FOODS TO REPLACE SUGAR TREATS		
fruit slices	vegetable sticks	granola
pretzels	salads	yogurt*
popcorn	almonds	peanuts
rice cakes	almond butter	peanut butter
mixed nuts	sunflower seeds	Protein smoothies
	pumpkin seeds	

* Plain yogurt without the sweeteners is a healthful snack. Fresh fruit can be added along with seasonings such as vanilla, cinnamon, or nutmeg.

A diet that is rich in whole grains and other complex carbohydrates, vegetables, and protein foods can also help stabilize blood sugar and minimize the desire for sugar. Many people who are protein-deficient seem to crave sugars and carbohydrate foods. Conversely, eating a diet that focuses on protein and vegetables is a good way to minimize sugar cravings. If handling sweets is a problem, fruits should be minimized and fruit juice avoided.

Nutrients that can help reduce the sugar craving and the symptoms of sugar withdrawal are the B vitamins, vitamin C, zinc, the trace mineral chromium, and the amino acid L-glutamine. Chromium is the central molecule of glucose, which helps insulin work more efficiently in removing sugar from the blood and nourishing the cells. The amino acid L-glutamine, which can be used directly by the brain, is also helpful in reducing sugar (and alcohol) cravings.

Children can also benefit from a nutritional supplement program which includes some of the above mentioned nutrients, of course in lower dosages than for adults. Use of a good quality children's multi-vitamin/mineral, additional B vitamins to support the nervous system and general development, vitamin C at about 250mg twice daily, and extra chromium all help to minimize sugar cravings and to transition from sugar and sweetened foods. The supplement plan for children applies to ages 6-11; amounts may vary from less to more depending on the age and size of each child. These vitamins are water soluble and basically nontoxic. However, if your child has a special problem or is below the age of six, you should check with your pediatrician or health-care provider for specific recommendations.

The use of sugar in our culture sometimes resembles use of a drug, and can be treated as such. Make a clear plan for withdrawal, while working emotionally to eliminate the habit. Responses to flavors, certain food compulsions, and the feelings we get from them are usually conditioned. Self-reflection can be valuable. To change our habits, to stop and see things clearly, or to talk them through helps us transition from compulsion to the safe and balanced use of foods, sugar, and sweetened foods, as well as other substances we may use in our life.

OVERCOMING A SWEET TOOTH

1. Take sugar overconsumption seriously—it can have insidious negative effects over time. This is particularly true for young people later in their lives.

2. Eat a diet which includes vegetables, whole grains (complex carbohydrates), and protein. Increasing protein levels in the diet, both animal and vegetable, helps to reduce sugar cravings and use.

3. If you seriously overuse sugar, omit it and consciously limit your intake of "hidden sweeteners" (particularly refined sugar (sucrose), corn syrup, and dextrose), and limit your use of honey and maple syrup. Eat some fruit, if you tolerate it, for natural sugar.

4. Support your body with extra helpful nutrients—these include the B vitamins, vitamin C, chromium, calcium, magnesium, and the amino acid L-glutamine.

5. Drink 6 to 8 glasses of water or herb tea a day.

6. Get sufficient fiber to keep your body cleansed and light.

7. If you suspect that you are hypoglycemic or diabetic, request the appropriate tests—such as a fasting blood sugar or a 5- or 6-hour glucose tolerance test—from your health care practitioner.

SUGAR DETOXIFICATION NUTRIENT PROGRAM

	ADULTS	CHILDREN
Water	2–3 qt	1-2 qt
Fiber	20–40 g	10-20 g
Vitamin E	200–800 IU	50-100 IU
Thiamine (B_1)	25–100 mg	10-50 mg
Riboflavin (B_2)	25–100 mg	10-25 mg
Niacinamide (B_3)	50–100 mg	10-50 mg
Pantothenic acid (B_5)	250–1,000 mg	50-250 mg
Pyridoxine (B_6)	25–100 mg	10-25 mg
Cobalamin (B_{12})	100–250 mcg	25-100 mcg
Folic acid	400-800 mcg	200-400 mcg
Vitamin C	2–10 g	500-1,000 mg
Bioflavonoids	250–500 mg	100-250 mg
Calcium	650–1,200 mg	350-600 mg
Chromium	200–500 mcg	100-250 mcg
Magnesium	400–800 mg	200-400 mg
Manganese	5–10 mg	3-5 mg
Selenium	200–300 mcg	50-100 mcg
Vanadium	200–400 mcg	50-150 mcg
Zinc	30–60 mg	15-30 mg
L-amino acids	1,000-1,500 mg	0
L-glutamine	500–1,000 mg	0
Essential fatty acids,	2–4 capsules	0
or Flaxseed oil	2–4 teaspoons	1-2 capsules
Adrenal glandular	100-200-mg	0

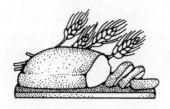

CHAPTER SIX

Drug Detoxification

Drug detoxification involves two main processes—changing our abusive habits and releasing the drugs from our bodies and our bodies and our lives.

We are a drug culture, and Western medicine is likewise a drug-oriented system. We consume billions of pills yearly and spend many billions of dollars buying them. These figures do not even begin to include the everyday use of caffeine, alcohol, and nicotine. There are really no stereotypical drug addicts. Affluent or poor people, anyone under pressure or with unmet psychological needs can end up with this problem. Substance abuse is an individual, family, and worldwide problem that can affect young and old, men and women.

It is important to understand the relationship between states of being, symptoms, and our use of drugs. In other words, if we view a symptom as problematic, we want to correct it with drugs. Although for immediate relief this may seem practical, it is theoretically short-sighted and shows a complete misunderstanding of human body design. In actuality, drug use and drug therapy rarely fix anything. Our symptoms serve as a warning sign of some bigger problem for which we must determine the cause. Symptoms are not the real problem, but rather are the results of deeper processes and causes. They are also not errors on the part of our body since our body rarely errs; rather, our body responds to the way we treat it. To correct aggravating symptoms, we must correct our internal imbalances and usually alter our lives. It is very important not to devitalize our body in any way if we can possibly avoid it. Since much habitual drug use is part of a syndrome of self-destruction, the first step for many people is to learn to care for and love themselves again, reinforcing their desire to live.

Pharmaceutical prescriptions and most over-the-counter (OTC) drugs are designed to help us feel better, yet they are too often used to treat problems resulting from abusive or misguided habits. This may aggravate the original problem or cause side effects. The promotion of addictions (which both support and drain our economy) begins with an emphasis on sugar. In fact, the use of sugar is so pervasive in our culture that it is difficult to find prepared or packaged foods that do not contain sugar or other sweeteners. Our habitual sweet tooth progresses to addictive usage of caffeine, nicotine, alcohol, and foods such as wheat, refined foods, and milk products. Later, the coffee break (combined with sugary snacks or coffee sweeteners) becomes a reward—a refueling rest stop during the workday. Caffeine and sugar stimulate us to work more. Nervousness and hyperactivity are often associated with productivity, although they are really not comparable to steady, healthful energy. Trying to perpetuate that productivity through the use of artificial stimulants eventually leads to reduced capacity, time lost from work, wasted money, and increased illness. Our behavior regarding foods, particularly sweet ones, is conditioned very early and is very difficult to change.

All drugs have some toxicity. Most have both physiological and psychological actions and addictive potential which result in accumulated toxicity and withdrawal symptoms when we try to give them up. Before going through any drug or chemical detoxification, it is wise to prepare for it. This is important both physically and psychologically, and it is definitely helpful to have a physician or other healthcare provider, therapist or counselor, family member or good friend for support. The withdrawal phase poses the most difficulties, and can last from a day or two to a week or more. It is often hard to differentiate the physical sensations from the underlying psychological involvement. The withdrawal phase itself is part of the drug addiction cycle—in other words, the worse the withdrawal, the more likely we are to continue to use the chemical to prevent those symptoms. A psychological dependency easily develops from the physical dependency.

After the initial withdrawal, where we detoxify through the release of stored chemicals from the body, we need willpower and commitment to keep the particular substance out of our life. We also need to work on new behavior patterns, such as avoiding exposure to the people and places associated with our previous problem until we develop new habits. Those new habits need to be strong enough so that we can easily say no when we are exposed to the substance again. Behavior modification therapy can be very helpful.

Characteristics of addiction include needing the drug to function, needing it in ever higher doses, needing it more frequently, feeling sick when a dose is missed, and/or having a history of abuse or addiction. The most useful approach to dealing with drug addiction begins with admitting that there is a problem. We must then combine our desire and willpower to accomplish this difficult task, and there are many support programs and government resources to help (see Resources, page 127). This decision often arises during illness or crisis rather than as a true desire to be healthy. Nonetheless, whatever gets us there is just fine—as long as we have the determination to follow through and stay on the path.

A well-balanced diet and nutritional supplements are essential to an effective plan, as is some psychological support. During the transition, either a cleansing diet or a fast is helpful to enhance purification and lessen the severity and length of withdrawal. I have seen people make dramatic lifestyle changes with only a week-long cleanse. Their new sense of empowerment helps them to clarify their goals while reinforcing their willpower.

The Detox Diet, which focuses primarily on steamed vegetables with some additional fruit and grains, allows a smooth transition with minimal withdrawal. It works to increase alkalinity and reduce acidity, which supports natural detoxification. Cravings and withdrawal intensify with an acid state generated by meats, milk products, and refined flours and sugars. A general diet with fruits and vegetables, juices and soups, or even water can be used temporarily, as they are alkaline-forming.

I do not suggest withdrawing or detoxifying from drugs during illness or either before or after surgery, although sometimes it is unavoidable. However, during pregnancy (ideally before pregnancy), it is important to clear all unnecessary drugs including OTC drugs, alcohol, nicotine, and caffeine. In all cases, we must be careful when withdrawing from these substances, although usually the basic daily habits can be tapered off and eliminated over the course of a few days. Since fetal stability is vitally important, it would be wise to have medical supervision during any form of detoxification during pregnancy.

Supplemental nutrients also support the system during drug elimination. Vitamin C and the other antioxidants—vitamins A and E, zinc and selenium, L-cysteine and other amino acids—are particularly important, in addition to a basic vitamin and mineral supplement. Glutathione, which is formed from L-cysteine in the body, acts in detoxification enzymes and helps decrease the toxicity of most drugs and chemicals.

A nutritional supplement approach to drug detoxification includes the B vitamins, minerals, a high amount of vitamin C, antioxidants, and the L- amino acids. These are more efficient when combined with a food diet than with fasting, and thus the alkaline, fruit- and vegetable-based diet is a better complement to any high nutrient intake. With a more liquid diet, I suggest minimizing your intake of supplements and recommend mainly vitamin C, some minerals, and an antioxidant formula, along with herbs and chlorophyll or algae products.

Herbal therapies can also be helpful. Goldenseal root powder is probably the most important herb as it not only stimulates the liver to better perform its detox function but also helps clear toxicity with its alkaloids. I usually suggest one large or two small capsules three times daily before meals for one or two weeks. Milk thistle, specifically *Silybum marianum*, also protects the liver from toxins and supports the detoxification process. Other helpful herbs during drug detoxification are those that work as laxatives, diuretics, and blood or lymph cleansers. Valerian root and other tranquilizing herbs may also lessen excitatory withdrawal symptoms such as anxiety or insomnia. Chlorophyll, taken as tablets or liquid, has a mildly purifying and rejuvenating quality.

Pharmaceuticals—Prescription and OTC Drugs

Any prescription or OTC drug can be toxic, especially when used too much or for too long. Aspirin, anti-inflammatory and pain-relieving drugs, tranquilizers, and anti-depressants are all in common use and are all similarly toxic, especially to the gastrointestinal tract.

The key to preventing the need to detoxify from drugs is to avoid their use in the first place. Many people are turning from Western medicine to alternative therapies and remedies as better preparation and knowledge has improved their efficacy. When used correctly, they support our body's natural healing powers and correct imbalances. Consult with a knowledgeable practitioner or information source for appropriate guidance, as herbs and other natural remedies (such as homeopathy) can produce occasional side effects as well. Acupuncture, osteopathic and chiropractic therapies, massage, and other body work can stimulate elimination and natural healing during detoxification periods.

Although OTC products are usually less toxic than pharmaceuticals, they are also more frequently abused as they can be readily obtained and are less expensive than most prescription drugs. Many symptoms are commonly treated with specific OTC drugs, seen in the as following chart.

COMMON OVER-THE-COUNTER (OTC) DRUGS	
Symptoms	**Drugs**
headache	aspirin, acetaminophen, ibuprofen
fatigue	caffeine, nicotine, No-Doz
insomnia	tranquilizers, antihistamines
colds, flus	antihistamines, decongestants
allergies	antihistamines, decongestants
constipation	laxatives, lubricants
diarrhea	Kaopectate, fibers
indigestion	antacids, Pepto-Bismol, Alka-Seltzer
excess weight	stimulants

Even at low potencies, many of these OTC drugs can create physical dependency. This is true especially when there is a chronic problem which requires long-term usage, or when there are withdrawal or rebound symptoms. If problems persist we should consult our healthcare practitioner to help us determine the underlying cause and work to correct that rather than continue to treat the symptoms alone. If stress and worry are the cause of insomnia or if poor food choices or meal times lead to our gastrointestinal symptoms, we need to make some lifestyle changes. If the symptoms persist, herbs or homeopathy are more gentle remedies.

Aspirin and caffeine are at the top of the OTC drug problems list. (Caffeine will be discussed thoroughly in the next chapter.) Aspirin, a valuable medicine in common use for many decades, is on the decline due to GI irritation and other concerns. Acetaminophen and other anti-inflammatory drugs have reduced the overall intake of aspirin. Still, acetylsalicylic acid (aspirin), derived from coal tar, has over 50 million regular users in this country consuming 20 to 25 billion tablets each year. Aspirin formulas often contain caffeine and act as anti-inflammatory agents. Aspirin works to reduce fevers (which, if left alone, are natural healers), and tends to work better than its counterpart acetaminophen (Tylenol, Datril). Both drugs are now in common use as people experience more pain and more degenerative conditions, such as cardiovascular disease. Low doses of aspirin have been found to reduce blood clotting effects.

The key to eliminating anti-inflammatory drugs is to eliminate the pain for which they are taken. Stronger pain drugs include the new anti-inflammatories such as ibuprofen (Medipren, Motrin), a drug with many side effects. Pain problems are frequently treated with even stronger prescription narcotics, such as codeine (aspirin or aceta-minophen with codeine is very commonly used), hydrocodone (Vicodin, Percodan), propoxyphene (Darvon), or even Demerol or morphine. All of these narcotic drugs are much more addictive, and thus more difficult to stop using.

Transition from Drugs to Natural Therapies

I began studying and working with natural medicines only after I learned about and was prescribing pharmaceutical drugs. Upon investigation, I became aware that many of the drugs I was prescribing had their basis or origin in plants. Some examples are Valium from valerian root, Ipecac from ipecaquana root, and digitalis from the foxglove plant. Scientists studied the active plant ingredients and then synthesized like molecules and stronger variations of those phytochemicals.

Well, I think we lost something in the transition—namely the safety and general positive effects with minimal side effects. We gained something also—power and speed. These drugs have greater, though sometimes more limited, effects, and of course, they usually have side effects and potential toxicity.

Over the last two decades, I have taken a back-to-nature approach. That means living more closely to and with greater reverence for Nature, and thus paying closer attention to how I live. I eat more wholesomely and I try to exercise and relax outdoors as often as possible. I have come to the awareness that my body is a part of Nature, not separate from her. After twenty years of finely tuning this awareness, I have learned to sense the subtlest adverse changes in my body. Since they are more subtle and less symptomatic, I can correct them with less invasive and safer therapies, specifically dietary changes, nutritional supplements, herbal and homeopathic remedies, body work, and hands-on therapies.

I encourage you to try a natural remedy the next time you experience a problem, unless of course, you believe your condition to be serious or dangerous. Some common examples of natural therapies include:

- **Fatigue**—rest, breathe, nature, massage, nutritional supplements, ginseng and other herbs
- **Insomnia**—exercise, calcium and magnesium, valerian root and other herbs, melatonin
- **Headache**—rest, water, detox, walk on the beach, white willowbark
- **Colds or Flu**—sleep, fluids, vitamins C and A, echinacea, goldenseal root

- **Constipation**—water, fiber, fruits and vegetables, abdominal massage, laxative herbs
- **Indigestion**—water and herb teas like peppermint, chamomile or licorice root, aloe vera juice, activated charcoal, assess for parasites
- **Allergies**—water, detox and juicing, vitamin C, and quercitin

One of the most exciting and rewarding aspects of my "natural-first" medical practice is the positive results my patients experience with minimal or no side effects. Over the years, they've discovered for themselves that eating well and exercising regularly removes the need to even consider taking drugs because they don't get sick! (Of course, if someone is acutely ill and/or in danger medically, I will use the quicker and stronger medications, and then later work to transition them to a more natural therapy.)

Please realize that all treatments—be they dietary changes, nutritional supplements and herbs, or drugs—are an experiment, or more accurately, an experience. Until you try them yourself, you cannot really know their exact affect upon your symptoms, disease, or health. To properly assess this personal experiment, be patient and be aware of and attentive to changes that occur. Initially, you may experience some adverse or unusual side effects, as in cleansing or healing reactions, but these should pass relatively quickly. (This is discussed more thoroughly in Chapters 2 and 10.)

More commonly (and importantly), there are many positive side effects and healthful rewards to using natural therapies. Patients often report feeling clear headed, physically energized, spiritually rejuvenated, and ready to set new goals and make new commitments. They look and feel younger, and have a vital, new sense of self with a more expansive and connected understanding. The key is to give Nature a chance. After all, you didn't accumulate the excess weight, poor digestion, ill health, or addictive habits overnight.

Other Drugs—Street and Recreational

Street or "recreational" narcotics are also a major social problem and generally pose a greater (though not insurmountable) challenge to detoxification. These include opium, methadone, heroin, and more recently "ice," and "crack." Heroin alone has over half a million addicted users. The drug creates a mix of euphoria and depression and also reduces the appetite and libido; food, sex, love, and nurturing often lose importance, and users' lives become focused upon obtaining and ingesting the drug.

Sleeping pills, tranquilizers, and antidepressants are also frequently used to replace dealing with life's frustrations and challenges. Valium was once the number one choice, but new drugs such as Ativan, Xanax, and Halcion are gaining in popularity. (Barbiturates used to be the main sedative but are now more frequently found on the street.) These drugs deal with anxiety by depressing our nervous system in a way somewhat like alcohol does, so I suggest using the principles and protocol described in the Alcohol chapter if these drugs are used.

Stimulants such as amphetamines and cocaine can cause dramatic fluctuations in energy. They excite the nervous system and promote euphoria or irritability but result in a loss of appetite, hypersensitivity, and insomnia, usually followed by fatigue and depression. The amphetamines (Dexedrine, Benzedrine, methamphetamine, and Desoxyn) are somewhat less popular than they were in prior years (probably because there are now better ways of getting high or losing weight), yet they remain a problem for some. As with the narcotics, amphetamine withdrawal and detoxification often require professional assistance, although some people manage it on their own. The stimulant drugs in general are more deadly than others, so it is very important to eliminate them if we want to live healthfully.

Again, stopping drugs can be dangerous. Going "cold turkey" from sedatives, stimulants, and narcotics can have very serious consequences, including seizures. There are many doctors and facilities, including hospital detox centers, available to help us deal with drug problems. The discussion of and specific treatments for drug abuse are beyond the scope of this book. Many of the suggestions in this text, specifically the Detox Diet and Nutritional Supplement guidelines, however, can be very useful in the process of detoxifying from such destructive habits.

The following program is intended as a supplement to a medical drug detoxification program and as support during necessary drug use. The ranges given allow for varying needs. During initial withdrawal, the higher levels should be used, with mid-range levels used during the three to six weeks directly following initial withdrawal. Lower ranges may provide basic support during general drug use.

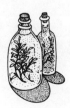

DRUG DETOXIFICATION NUTRIENT PROGRAM

Water	2–3 1/2 qt	Bioflavonoids	250–500 mg
Fiber	20–40 g	Calcium	650–1,200 mg+
Vitamin A	5,000-10,000 IU	Chromium	200–500 mcg
Beta-carotene	20,000–40,000 IU	Copper	2–3 mg
Vitamin D	200–400 IU	Iodine	150 mcg
Vitamin E	200–800 IU	Iron	10–20 mg**
Vitamin K	300 mcg	Magnesium	400–800 mg+
Thiamine (B$_1$)	25–100 mg	Manganese	5–10 mg
Riboflavin (B$_2$)	25–100 mg	Molybdenum	150–300 mcg
Niacinamide (B$_3$)	50–100 mg	Potassium	100–500 mg
Niacin (B$_3$)	50–1,000 mg*	Selenium	200–300 mcg
Pantothenic acid (B$_5$)	250–1,000 mg	Silicon	50–150 mg
Pyridoxine (B$_6$)	25–100 mg	Vanadium	200–400 mcg
Pyridoxal-5-phosphate	25–50 mg	Zinc	30–60 mg
Cobalamin (B$_{12}$)	100–250 mcg	L-amino acids	1,000-1,500 mg
Folic acid	800 mcg	L-cysteine	250–500 mg
Biotin	300 mcg	L-glutamine	250–1,000 mg
Choline	500–1,000 mg	Essential fatty acids	2–4 capsules
Inositol	500–1,000 mg	Flaxseed oil	2–4 teaspoons
Vitamin C	2–10 g	Goldenseal root	3–6 capsules

* Increase dosage slowly.
** As needed if low.
\+ Higher amounts are needed for hyperactive withdrawal states, aches, or cravings.

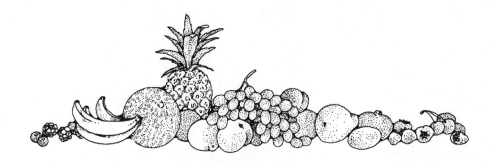

DRUG DETOX SUMMARY

1. Drink plenty of water and consider the Detox Diet to help you transition from your habit.

2. If you are a heavy drug user, use the assistance of a health care practitioner to support your detox. Going "cold turkey" from sedatives, stimulants, and narcotics can have very serious consequences, including seizures.

3. If you are pregnant, use medical supervision to stop using drugs. Acupuncture has a particularly good reputation for helping moms detox and supporting full-term, healthy babies.

4. Reduce stress in your life. Enhance your coping strategies and support systems.

5. Use psychological supports which fit your value system: counseling, biofeedback, DA (Drugs Anonymous), or behavior modification.

6. Use supplemental nutrients to support your body during detox. Include regular vitamin C, B vitamins, and most minerals, particularly calcium and magnesium for their calming effects.

7. Try herbal therapies to ease the detox process—white willow bark for pains, valerian root and others for anxiety and insomnia. If these are not strong enough, prescription medications can be used temporarily to help ease withdrawal.

8. Consider the use of acupuncture and Chinese herbal therapy to ease the body through its transition.

CHAPTER SEVEN

Caffeine Detoxification

◆

Caffeine has become a ubiquitous drug. Used originally in most cultures for ceremonies, it has become an overused energy stimulant in the Western world with the United States leading in coffee and caffeine use.

Coffee, brewed from the ground coffee bean (*Coffea arabica*), is the major vehicle for caffeine consumption. In this country, more than a half billion cups are consumed daily, with most people drinking two or more cups a day. More than ten pounds of coffee per person are consumed yearly. This food/drug mixture—often combined with sugar and/or milk—is one of the most freely marketed addictive substances in the world.

There are several basic areas of concern, not the least of which focuses on the toxic chemicals used in growing and processing coffee. The easily rancified oils and the irritating acids contained in the beans themselves offer further hazards. People trying to cut down by drinking decaffeinated coffee could be exposed to even more dangerous chemicals unless they are drinking water-processed decaf. This Swiss process uses steam distillation to remove the caffeine whereas regular decaffeination uses agents such as TCE (trichlorethylene) or methylene chloride which leave residues in the prepared decaf coffee itself. The last few decades have also seen an increase in the use of pesticides and chemical processing.

In 1946—the peak of US coffee use—yearly consumption was 20 pounds per person. Since most children and some adults were not consuming any coffee, many people in 1946 were consuming more than the 1,000-cup-a-year average. From 1980 to 1990, coffee consumption averaged about 10 pounds a year (US Department of Agriculture, annual statistics). Slight drops were reported in consumption from 1990-1993.

Two trends are evident related to beverage intake: people are developing healthier habits by drinking more light fruit juices, fresh vegetables juices, and water. From 1980 to 1993, the average intake of bottled water increased from 2.4 to 9.2 gallons.

Yet, coffee consumption may be on the rise, as social events increasingly include fashionable coffee beverages such as espresso, cappuccino, and lattes.

Another problem is caffeine's widespread use as an ingredient in so many products, including some soft drinks and many OTC drugs. The problem here is less with the drug itself and more with the amounts consumed and the constant stimulation on which people come to depend many times daily, sometimes unknowingly. One big area of concern here is with children and teenagers, who may consume large amounts of caffeine when drinking soft drinks. Cola naturally contains caffeine, yet many soft drinks have additional amounts which promote an addiction to the drink. Cocoa, which also contains caffeine, has become more popular in the United States. Consumption has increased from approximately 4 pounds per person in 1970 to 5.4 pounds per person in 1990, and 5.8 pounds per person in 1993.

Another concern is that caffeine is often consumed along with other substances such as nicotine and sugar. Like sugar, caffeine overstimulates the adrenals and then weakens them with persistent or chronic use. A cycle develops where first sugar stimulates and weakens the adrenals, creating fatigue to which we then respond by drinking caffeine to stay awake. In addition, people who overuse caffeine tend to need more tranquilizers and sleeping pills to help them relax or sleep. Caffeine is a lifetime drug for many. We begin at a young age with hot chocolate or chocolate bars, move into colas or other soft drinks, and then add coffee and tea.

Physiologically, caffeine is a central nervous system (CNS) stimulant. It is a member of the class of methylxanthine chemicals/drugs. Xanthines (specifically theophylline) are commonly used in medicine to aid in breathing. Theobromine, another xanthine derivative, is found in cocoa. Methylxanthines are found in many other plants, including the kola nut originally used to make cola drinks. A dosage of 50–100 mg caffeine, the amount in one cup of coffee, will produce a temporary increase in mental clarity and energy levels while simultaneously reducing drowsiness. It also improves muscular-coordinated work activity, such as typing. Through its CNS stimulation, caffeine increases brain activity; however it also stimulates the cardiovascular system, raising blood pressure and heart rate. It generally speeds up our body by increasing our basal metabolic rate (BMR), which burns more calories. Initially, caffeine may lower blood sugar; however, this can lead to increased hunger or cravings for sweets. After adrenal stimulation, blood sugar rises again. Caffeine also increases respiratory rates, and for people with tight airways, it can open breathing passages (as do the other xanthine drugs). Caffeine is also a diuretic and a mild laxative.

The amount of caffeine needed to produce stimulation increases with regular use, as is typical of all addictive drugs. Larger and more frequent doses are needed to achieve the original effect, and symptoms can develop if we do not get our "fix." Eventually, we need the drug to function; without it, fatigue, drowsiness, and headaches can occur.

Unfortunately, most caffeine products do not contain any of the nutrients, such as manganese and copper, needed to support the increased activity that they cause. Also, the diuretic effect of caffeine leads to the urinary loss of many nutrients which frequently go unreplaced.

Overall, addiction to caffeine is not as bad as addiction to most other drugs. Usually, the slower the tapering of use, the easier the withdrawal. After complete withdrawal and detoxification from caffeine, it is possible to use it in moderation, but care must be taken as it can be re-addicting.

SIGNS AND SYMPTOMS OF CAFFEINE INTOXICATION OR ABUSE

nervousness	headache	increased heart rate
anxiety	upset stomach	irregular heartbeat
irritability	GI irritation	elevated blood pressure
agitation	heartburn	increased cholesterol
tremors	diarrhea	nutritional deficiencies
insomnia	fatigue	poor concentration
depression	dizziness	bed wetting

CAFFEINE WITHDRAWAL SYMPTOMS

headache	anxiety	vomiting
craving	nervousness	cramps
irritability	shakiness	ringing in the ears
insomnia	dizziness	feeling hot and cold
fatigue	drowsiness	tachycardia
depression	inability to concentrate	
apathy	runny nose	
constipation	nausea	

The most common caffeine withdrawal symptom is a throbbing and/or pressure headache, usually located at the temples but occasionally at the back of the head or around the eyes. A vague muscular headache often follows. Of course, caffeine can cure these symptoms; but this is not the answer. Rather, we need to adhere to dietary guidelines and supplements to help with this and other withdrawal problems. It is best to taper off caffeine before going on a cleanse as the withdrawal (mainly headaches) can be very uncomfortable. The Detox Diet works well for this transition.

Coffee is not the only product in our diet that contains caffeine. Of the teas, all black or common teas such as Earl Grey or English Breakfast contain theophylline and theobromine, as do some green teas. Both contain less caffeine than coffee. Tannic acid, a mild irritant to the gastrointestinal mucosa which may reduce absorption of minerals such as manganese, zinc, and copper can be found in both coffee and tea. Most herbs do not contain caffeine, although maté and guarana are fairly high in caffeine. The kola nut and the cocoa bean also contain caffeine. Ephedra or mahuang is a Chinese herb that gives caffeine-like stimulation. These natural products have been used as stimulants throughout history.

Both extracted and synthesized caffeine may be added to other products. Many common pharmaceutical preparations contain caffeine for its stimulating effects which counteract the sedating antihistamines, or for its cerebral vasodilating effects used to relieve vascular headaches. Cafergot is a prescription drug containing caffeine and is used for migraines; although caffeine can help reduce headaches, it more commonly causes them.

CAFFEINE DRUGS AVAILABLE OVER THE COUNTER

Stimulants—NoDoz, Vivarin, Refresh'n

Weight control—Dexatrim, Dietac

Pain Relief—Excedrin, Anacin, Vanquish, Empirin Compound

Menstrual pain relief—Midol, Premens, Aqua-Ban, Cope

Cold remedies—Dristan, Sinarest

Caffeine, although it is not seriously addicting, is very habit forming. Anyone interested in high-level health should avoid it. Although it may improve short-term performance, it eventually creates long-term depletion.

CAFFEINE LEVELS* IN COMMON SUBSTANCES**

Coffee and Other Drinks/6 oz cup	Amount of Caffeine (mg)
Drip	120-150
Percolated	80-110
Instant	60-70
Decaf	3-10
Espresso (1 oz shot)	75
Caffe Latte	70
Cappuccino	70
Caffe Mocha	80
Black tea	50-60
Earl Grey	50
English Breakfast	50
Green tea	30-40
Jasmine	20
Cocoa	10-30
Chocolate milk	10-15
Cocoa (dry, 1 oz.)	40-50
Chocolate (dry, 1 oz.)	5-10

Soft drink, per 12 oz. serving	
Colas	30-65
Mountain Dew	50

OTC Medicines	
NoDoz	100
Vivarin	200
Dexatrim	200
Dietac	200
Cafergot	100
Excedrin	65
Fiorinal	40
Anacin	30
Vanquish	35
Aqua-Ban	100
Midol	30

* These caffeine levels and caffeine equivalents may depend on length of brewing time or amount of product used. The levels given are approximate.

** Information gathered and integrated from at least six different sources.

Negative Effects of Caffeine

Most of the negative effects of caffeine are not a concern with occasional use, but can occur with regular use of over 100 mg daily. The risks discussed in the following list vary with the level of caffeine intake and individual sensitivity. A total of over 500 mg caffeine daily is a high intake, and the total includes all coffee, tea, soft drinks, and drugs. Between 250 and 500 mg might be classified as moderate intake, while under 250 mg would be low. For a long time, the popularity of caffeine outweighed its negative effects. Now the dangers are fairly clear, and it is hard to refute the evidence. Common negative effects include:

- excess nervousness, irritability, insomnia, "restless legs," dizziness, and subsequent fatigue
- headaches
- "heartburn"
- general anxiety (even panic attacks)
- hyperactivity and bed wetting in children who consume caffeine
- increased stomach hydrochloric acid production (clearly bad for people with existing ulcers or gastritis)
- loss of minerals such as potassium, magnesium, and zinc, and vitamins including the B vitamins, particularly thiamine and vitamin C
- reduced absorption of iron and calcium (especially when caffeine is consumed around mealtime)
- osteoporosis and anemia
- interrupted growth in children and adolescents
- diarrhea
- increased blood pressure and hypertension, especially in atherosclerosis and heart disease
- increased cholesterol and triglyceride blood levels
- heart rhythm disturbances and mild arrythmias, tachycardia, and palpitations
- increased norepinephrine secretion, which causes some vasoconstriction (although caffeine may have mild vasodilating effects in the heart and body, excess adrenal stimulation may override this)
- increased risk of heart attacks (while results are mixed, it seems reasonable to assume that drinking four to five cups of coffee per day does increase the incidence of myocardial infarctions due to cardiovascular stimulation)

- fibrocystic breast disease (again, results vary, but it is clear that some women experience an increase in size and number of cysts with increased use of caffeine)
- birth defects and spontaneous abortions (caffeine does cross the placenta and affects the fetus, but the distinct cause of mutagenic effects is not clear. It is wise to limit or completely avoid the use of caffeine during pregnancy and lactation.)
- kidney stones, which can occur as a result of the diuretic and chemical effects
- increased fevers, both as a direct effect and by counteracting the effect of aspirin
- increased incidence of certain cancers including bladder cancer (more frequently due to a combination with nicotine), ovarian cancer and pancreatic cancer
- prostate enlargement may also be attributed to increased caffeine intake
- the adrenal exhaustion/stress/fatigue/hypoglycemia syndrome is tied to caffeine use. While caffeine has the overall effect of increasing blood sugar, stress and sugar intake weaken the adrenal function. Recovery from the resulting fatigue requires rest, stress reduction, and sugar avoidance, and even though caffeine can override this fatigue and restimulate the adrenals temporarily, eventually chronic fatigue, adrenal exhaustion, and subsequent inability to handle any stress or sugar will result. Caffeine will *then* be of little help.

Detoxification from Caffeine

Anyone with a regular caffeine habit should seriously consider discontinuing its use until they can reach a state of occasional enjoyment. If addiction is clear, or in cases of pregnancy, caffeine should given up completely. Breaking the habit by either tapering off or going "cold turkey" will be easier with a good diet and adrenal support.

Two or three weeks of the Detox Diet can support the transition into a healthier and caffeine-free program. The post-detox diet includes vegetable salads, soups, greens, seaweed, corn, some whole grains, sprouts, soy products, and some nuts and seeds, using fruit for snacks. A decreased intake of acid foods such as meat, sugar and refined flour is also a good idea, as is avoiding the overuse of baked goods (even whole grain products), nuts, and seeds. Drinking at least six to eight glasses of filtered water a day and sipping mineral water or herbal teas can help replace the coffee habit. Baking soda or, better, potassium bicarbonate tablets, will not only help make our bodies more alkaline but also reduce withdrawal symptoms.

Additionally, vitamin C supplementation helps during withdrawal by supporting the adrenal glands. As a stress-reducer, several grams or more of vitamin C can be taken over the course of the day, preferably in a buffered form, especially with minerals such as potassium, calcium, magnesium, and zinc. I also suggest B complex vitamins with extra pantothenic acid (250 mg four times daily), along with 500 mg of vitamin C every two or three hours.

During average coffee use, we need to be careful to replenish depleted nutrients including thiamine (B$_1$), riboflavin (B$_2$), pyridoxine (B$_6$), vitamin C, potassium, magnesium and, to a lesser degree, zinc, iron, calcium, and the trace minerals. Additional amino acids can help balance our energy level during use of or withdrawal from caffeine. Water intake and additional fiber will support bowel function, which frequently slows down during caffeine withdrawal.

Spreading the detoxification program over a week or two and reducing caffeine intake to none will help avoid significant headaches. Lower caffeine intake by drinking grain-coffee blends, diluted or smaller amounts of regular coffee, or decaffeinated coffee (water processed). Another approach is to first substitute black tea, which has less caffeine than coffee, and can be tapered off of more easily.

If headaches occur, mild pain relievers can be used for a few days, but avoid taking them over a longer period of time. Increased water intake, vitamin C and mineral support, an alkaline diet, and white willow bark herb tablets, which contain a natural salicylate, should ease these withdrawal symptoms.

There are a number of herbal teas to use in place of coffee that can be both stimulating and refreshing. The roasted herbal roots, including barley, chicory, and dandelion, are most popular. Grain "coffees," such as Postum, Pero, Cafix, Rombouts, and Wilson's Heritage, are also favored among former coffee drinkers, while ginseng root tea is preferred by some. The Chinese herb ephedra acts as a stimulant and can be used during the transition from caffeine, although I do not recommend regular intake, as its stimulating properties can be weakening over time. Herbal teas made from lemon grass, peppermint, ginger root, red clover, and comfrey are very nourishing, and do not have the depleting side effects. The algaes can also be energizing in place of caffeine.

If we do drink a cup of coffee or caffeinated tea a day, we should do so in the mid to late afternoon. This best fits our body's natural cycle, avoiding the high-adrenal morning and late pre-sleep hours. Those who cannot relax or sleep well after using caffeine should consider avoiding it altogether.

The pleasures of coffee and tea drinking are as much a cultural phenomenon as they are a taste preference. Remember, habits are developed, not inherent, and anything we learn, we can also unlearn or relearn.

Use the lower ranges of nutrients in the following table for general support and the higher levels for detoxification. The amounts shown are daily totals, and should be divided into two or three supplementations during the day.

HERBAL CAFFEINE SUBSTITUTES

Roasted barley	Rostaroma	Ginger root
Chicory root	Wilson's Heritage	Ephedra
Dandelion root	Cafix	Comfrey leaf
Postum	Miso broth	Lemon grass
Pero	Duran	Red clover
Pioneer	Peppermint	Comfrey leaf
Rombouts	Ginseng root	Teeccino

CAFFEINE SUPPORT AND DETOX NUTRIENT PROGRAM

Water	2 1/2 –3 qt	Calcium	800–1,000 mg
Fiber	15–20 g	Chromium	200–400 mcg
Vitamin A	5,000-10,000 IU	Copper	2–3 mg
Beta-carotene	15,000-25,000 IU	Iodine	150 mcg
Vitamin D	400 IU	Iron*	
Vitamin E	400–800 IU	men	0–15 mg
Vitamin K	300 mcg	women	15–30 mg
Thiamine (B_1)	75–150 mg	Magnesium	500–800 mg
Riboflavin (B_2)	50–100 mg	Manganese	5–10 mg
Niacinamide (B_3)	50–100 mg	Molybdenum	300–500 mcg
Niacin (B_3)	50–100 mg	Potassium	300–600 mg
Pantothenic acid (B_5)	500–1,000 mg	Silicon	50–100 mg
Pyridoxine (B_6)	50–100 mg	Selenium	200–300 mcg
Pyridoxal-5-phosphate	25–50 mg	Zinc	30-60 mg
Cobalamin (B_{12})	100–200 mcg	Adrenal	50–150 mg
Folic acid	400–800 mcg	L-amino acids	500–1,500 mg
Biotin	300 mcg	Potassium bicarbonate**	600–1,000 mg
Vitamin C	2–6 g	Herbal teas	3 cups daily
Bioflavonoids	250–500 mg	Blue-green algae	500-2,000 mg.

 * Level would depend on lab values; otherwise, use only 10 mg/day maximum.
** Can use Alka-Seltzer Effervescent Antacid, one tablet 2–3 times daily.

CAFFEINE DETOX SUMMARY

1. If you take in more than 500 mg. a day of caffeine, consider taking a break from it, and clearing your body of caffeine. If you are pregnant and have high caffeine intake, detox under the guidance of a health care practitioner.

2. After that, avoid the daily use of caffeine. For most people, it can still be tolerated and enjoyed as long as it does not become a daily habit.

3. Consider the Detox Diet or a general alkaline diet consisting mainly of vegetables, both steamed and as salads, fruits, plus some whole grains, soy protein, and a few nuts or seeds.

4. Drink at least 6 to 8 glasses of water daily or more, especially if you exercise and sweat.

5. Keep fiber intake high to help clear the colon and support detoxification.

6. Supplement your nutrition with vitamins and minerals as outlined on facing page.

7. If headaches occur, as they commonly do in the first few days of detox, increase your intake of water, vitamin C, and minerals, and use white willow bark herb to ease headaches and withdrawal.

8. Other herbs, particularly as teas, can be taken to support the body or as coffee substitutes.

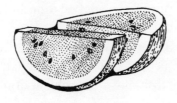

CHAPTER EIGHT

Alcohol Detoxification

Even though alcohol is enjoyed worldwide and has been used for thousands of years, its regular over-consumption poses a serious health hazard. As with caffeine, occasional or moderate use is often pleasurable and is no cause for concern except for people with allergic reactions to alcohol or diseases of the liver, gastrointestinal tract, kidneys, brain, or nervous system. Habitual alcohol over-consumption, however, can lead to addiction, emotional problems, and a number of specific degenerative processes including obesity, gastritis and ulcers, pancreatitis, hepatitis, cirrhosis, hypoglycemia and diabetes, gout, nerve and brain dysfunction, cancer, nutritional deficiencies, immune suppression, accidental injury, and death. Most people can handle periodic use, but for many others, it is a significant problem.

Alcohol does have some positive physiological effects. It stimulates the appetite and relieves stress, although not as much as exercise. It acts as a vasodilator, improving blood flow. Alcohol may also affect a slight increase in HDL "good" cholesterol levels, however it also raises total blood fats. Small to moderate amounts (one to two drinks daily) may also lessen the progression of atherosclerosis and heart disease. Some studies have shown a lower number of heart attacks in moderate drinkers over non-drinkers of the same age, possibly due to increased HDL cholesterol levels, and reduced atherosclerosis. Higher amounts of alcohol, however, increase blood pressure and heart disease risk. More research is needed to understand the real link between alcohol and heart disease before prescribing it as a preventative measure. Certainly regular physical activity and nurturing personal relationships are better health supporters and stress reducers than alcohol.

There are over 100 million regular drinkers in the United States alone and about 11 million who report heavy alcohol use. More than half of our population are social drinkers (138 million). Social drinking and problem drinking mean different things to different people. If you feel that alcohol is a problem for you, consider the following:

If you drink more than two drinks each evening or if you drink more than five times per week, you may want to look into changing your habit.

Alcohol is a particularly big concern for our youth. More and more children are trying alcohol, and in 1992, an estimated 5 percent of children ages 12-17 consumed alcohol more than 50 days during that year.

Empty Calories Mean Insufficient Nutrition

Alcohol is a source of empty calories; it contains seven of them per gram, almost double the calories found in regular carbohydrates and protein (four calories per gram each). The average social drinker consumes 5–10 percent of his or her calories from alcohol, while heavy drinkers may consume more than 50 percent in place of real nutrition. Since alcohol is replacing regular nutrition, the body receives decreased amounts of essential vitamins, minerals, and other nutrients, causing deficiencies over time. In addition, the alcohol molecule is so small and easy to absorb that it gets assimilated before other foods, directly entering the bloodstream for a quick effect. Beer, wine, and mixed drinks cause rapid fluctuations of the blood sugar with accompanying mood swings.

The liver is the only organ that metabolizes alcohol, either converting it into energy or storing it as fat when there is excess consumption. When stored as fat, alcohol acts as an irritant and can eventually lead to cirrhosis, or scarring of the liver tissue. About five percent of ingested alcohol is eliminated through sweat, urine, and breath.

Many people think of alcohol as a stimulant because it reduces inhibitions and, in small amounts, seems to ease and enhance social interactions. It is actually a sedative that depresses the central nervous system. The effects are pleasantly tranquilizing at first. However, with continued consumption the calming effect deteriorates into mental and physical numbness, hampering our reflexes, coordination, and judgment. This is why there are so many alcohol-related accidents both while walking and driving.

Despite all these problems, alcohol is rooted in our culture. For centuries alcohol was used as an anesthetic to treat physical pain. Nowadays it is used to anesthetize emotional pain. Alcohol abuse and alcoholism are clearly diseases which involve genetics, social/cultural values, and environmental influences and which have emotional consequences. It is possible that it may involve an enzyme deficiency, or be linked to a deficiency or improper function of chromium (a trace mineral related to blood sugar metabolism). Whatever its cause, problems related to alcohol abuse definitely seem to run in families.

Alcohol drinks can also be allergenic as they contain grains, grapes, sugar, and yeast producing both intestinal and cerebral symptoms. Corn, wheat, rye, and barley can also cause allergic reactions. Alcoholism may even be an advanced food addiction in which the allergens themselves stimulate addiction; in such cases, withdrawal from the offending food produces uncomfortable psychological and physical symptoms. Alcohol products are also problematic for people with a yeast overgrowth, as it feeds the yeast and stimulates its growth. Furthermore, many people react to various chemicals, such as sulfites, which are used in manufacturing alcohol.

It has been suggested that alcohol is a viable source of nourishment. Wine does contain vitamin C from grape or rice juice, yet it also contains 9–12 percent alcohol (empty calories). In sherry and port wines, alcohol content may be as high as 12–18 percent. Beers and ale contain B vitamins and minerals from the cereal grains and yeast, with a range from of 3–6 percent alcohol. Alcohol distillates or "spirits" such as gin, vodka, rum, and whiskey are also made from grain products. These range from 35–50 percent alcohol—that is, 70–100 proof. In reality, none of these beverages are very nourishing when calorie levels are compared to nutrient levels.

CALORIE CONTENT OF ALCOHOLIC BEVERAGES

Amount to Provide 0.5 oz of Alcohol	Type of Beverage	Calories
1 oz	100 or 110 proof liquor	80
1 1/2 oz	80 proof liquor	90–110
5 oz	8–10 percent wine (French, German)	100
4 oz	12–14 percent wine (most American)	95
3 oz	17–20 percent wine (sherry, port)	80
2 1/2 oz	18 percent dessert wine	120
8 oz	6–7 percent dark beer (stout, porter)	150
12 oz	4.5 percent regular beer	140
12 oz	light beer	90
6 oz	mixed drinks (various juices, sodas, sweeteners)	100–250

Risks of Alcohol

The risk levels of alcohol are directly related to the amount consumed and the time period over which it is used, although individual reactions may vary. High-risk use involves more than five drinks daily; moderate-risk use, three to five drinks daily; and low-risk, one or two. Social drinking of a few drinks a week offers minimal risk.

Those with diabetes, hypertension, or heart disease, and pregnant or nursing mothers, or those planning pregnancy should not drink alcohol at all. People with hypoglycemic problems, liver disorders (especially hepatitis), ulcers and gastritis, viral diseases, candidiasis, mental confusion, fatigue, or hypersensitive reactions to alcoholic beverages should also avoid it.

Symptoms from drinking include dizziness, delayed reflexes, slowed mental functions, memory loss, poor judgment, emotional outburst, aggressive behavior, lack of coordination, and loss of consciousness. **Symptoms of hangover** include mouth dryness, thirst, headache, throbbing temples, nausea, vomiting, stomach upset, fatigue, and dizziness. Alcohol dehydrates the cells, removes fluid from the blood, swells the cranial arteries, and irritates the gastrointestinal tract. Hangovers are more common with stronger, distilled alcohol drinks but can still occur with red and white wines, champagne, and beer.

Symptoms of withdrawal include alcohol craving, nausea, vomiting, gastrointestinal upset, abdominal cramps, anorexia, fatigue, headache, anxiety, irritability, dizziness, fevers, chills, depression, insomnia, tremors, weakness, hallucinations, and seizures.

Drinking can put us at risk to inadvertently harm ourselves or others. Alcohol is involved in the more than 25,000 **auto accidents deaths** yearly. About 20 percent of home **accidental deaths** are attributed to alcohol.

Ninety-five percent of alcohol consumed must be metabolized in the liver, taking precedence over other functions. Fat metabolism slows and fat builds up in the liver. Since alcohol converts to fat, **obesity** also often occurs with high alcohol use. Chronic use can swell, scar, and shrink the liver, until only a small percentage is functional. Complications also include ascites (fluid buildup in the abdomen), hemorrhoids, varicose veins, and bleeding disorders. More serious **liver disease** such as hepatitis and cirrhosis, when the liver becomes inflamed or enlarged, are also the result of chronic alcohol use. Usually more than half the liver must be destroyed before its work is significantly impaired (but it can regenerate if drinking is stopped).

Gastrointestinal disorders include gastritis, abdominal pain, eating difficulties, gastric ulcers, duodenal ulcers, deficiency of hydrochloric acid and digestive enzymes, "leaky gut" syndrome, esophagitis (irritation of the esophagus), varicose veins, pancreatitis, gallstones, and gall bladder disease.

Alcohol can cross the blood-brain barrier, destroying brain cells and causing brain damage and behavioral and psychological problems; **nervous system disorders,** including polyneuritis (nerve inflammations), premature senility, and encephalopathy (chronic degenerative brain syndrome) can also result from chronic alcohol use.

Although modest alcohol intake may, in fact, raise HDL cholesterol and protect against atherosclerosis, the effect of alcohol abuse on the heart and blood vessels is damaging and leads to **cardiovascular diseases and disfunctions.** These include a decrease in heart function, heart muscle action, and electrical conductivity, congestive heart failure, cardiac arrythmias, and an enlarged heart.

Carbohydrate metabolism is effected by alcohol and can lead to hypoglycemia and diabetes. Alcohol is a simple sugar that is rapidly absorbed and which has a tendency to weaken glucose tolerance with chronic use. Impaired glucose metabolism can cause mood swings, depression, emotional outbursts, or anxiety. Furthermore, increased calories from alcohol can lead to weight gain and increased body fat resulting in **obesity** as alcohol converts to fat unless it is balanced by exercise and a good diet.

Nutritional deficiencies from alcohol use include impaired absorption of nutrients, particularly B vitamins and minerals; liver impairment from reduced absorption of the fat-soluble vitamins A, D, E, and K; loss of nutrients from alcohol's diuretic effect; reduced liver stores of alcohol-metabolizing vitamins B_1 and B_3; anemia due to deficiency of folic acid, vitamin B_{12}, and iron; increased risk of osteoporosis from low vitamin D and poor calcium absorption; lack of appetite, causing deficiencies in vitamin B_2, B_6, A, C, essential fatty acid, and methionine.

Alcohol increases levels of the liver enzyme that breaks down testosterone. In teenage boys, the reduction of testosterone may delay sexual maturity. Alcohol's depressant effect on the nervous system **can reduce sexual performance** or cause **impotence** despite reduced inhibitions and increased desire.

Alcohol has been implicated in **malignancies** of the mouth, esophagus, pancreas, and breasts. Cigarette smoke and alcohol combined are thought to create ethyl nitrite, which is a strong mutagen. **Other health problems** include a red swollen nose, dilated blood vessels, gout, yeast vaginitis, PMS, and a suppressed immune system. Because alcohol crosses the placenta and enters fetal circulation, **fetal alcohol syndrome** results in undersized babies often with mental deficits due to brain damage. There is no "safe" level—women who are pregnant should simply not drink!

Regular alcohol use and abuse can create **social problems** in personal relationships and career, and economic adversity in regard to lost work and medical costs.

Alcoholism

The alcoholic is someone who has lost control over the drug. Research suggests that there is a genetic component to problem drinking. An intense biological craving for alcohol or the products from which it is made might be at the root, as might problems with blood sugar metabolism or allergy-addictions. The ability to easily stop drinking for a week or two at a time is a good sign. Remember, many people with a drinking problem deny that there is one. Warning signs of alcoholism include drinking alone, drinking in place of meals, drinking before social or business functions, drinking in the morning or late at night, missing work because of drinking, and periods of amnesia or blackouts. People who have these concerns should definitely seek help.

Once we've admitted that we need outside resources to deal with alcohol, it is important to get the support of our spouse or a friend. Clear the alcohol from all areas of life (home, work, car, etc.), and then see a physician or therapist. A medical check-up with laboratory testing may be in order. Some cases require tranquilizers during the first few days of withdrawal. With a multilevel approach combining community and professional support, the chances of recovery from alcohol are better than 50 percent.

Psychological counseling, family therapy, Alcoholics Anonymous (AA), or religious/spiritual practices may also improve our motivation, self-image, and ability to create a new life. AA meetings continue the positive support for many recovering alcoholics. Avoiding negative influences such as old drinking buddies and exposure to alcohol is also helpful. Regular exercise is valuable, especially at the usual drinking time. Additionally, weight training is an excellent way to work off stress and anger. Learning and practicing relaxation exercises can also be useful. Massage therapy promotes relaxation and self-love. Acupuncture is usually beneficial during withdrawal and detox, as it seems to reduce the stress from cravings that may reappear periodically after the initial detox process.

The amount of time it takes to detoxify from alcohol depends on the level of abuse, and it may take months or even years to completely clear its effects. Mild withdrawal symptoms include increased tension, headaches, and irritability for a few days. Medical care in a hospital setting is not uncommon for acute alcohol withdrawal, although this is usually necessary only for those who consume more than six to eight drinks daily.

If willpower is poor, drugs such as Antabuse (disulfiram), which produce terrible nausea and vomiting when alcohol is used, can be a powerful deterrent. Antabuse is usually fairly well tolerated for a short time, but it can have side effects on the cardio-vascular system and psyche. Lithium therapy has recently been shown to reduce the urge to drink. For recovering alcoholics, I believe that it is imperative to avoid all alcohol for life, because the addictive potential never disappears. Nonalcoholic beverages may be fine, but even some de-alcoholized drinks contain small amounts of the drug.

Alcohol Detoxification

Diet and megavitamin therapy are helpful during withdrawal, detoxification, and recovery. Certainly, people who use alcohol excessively need more supplements than others, and during detox they may require even more. During the actual withdrawal period, diet should focus on fluids and alkaline foods. The appetite is usually not active at this time; liquids are easy to consume and will also help clear alcohol from the body. Water, diluted fruit and vegetable juices, warm broths, soups, and teas using herbs such as chamomile, skullcap (a nervine), or valerian root are good choices. Other helpful herbs include white willow bark for reducing pain and inflammation, ginseng, cayenne, and peppermint. Small amounts of light proteins, such as nonfatty poultry, fish, or even chicken soup will provide more nourishment. Amino acid powder is also supportive. L-glutamine, an amino acid, has been shown to reduce cravings for alcohol and sugar, and is used in many detox clinics.

I have seen intravenous supplements work quite well during withdrawal. Extra vitamin C, B complex, and minerals such as calcium, magnesium, and potassium, can be used intravenously, especially if supplements taken by mouth are not well tolerated. Vitamin C powder buffered with these minerals and mixed into water or juice is helpful during withdrawal and later during the detox period.

Alcohol detoxification continues for several weeks after withdrawal. During this recovery time, the body will eliminate alcohol, its by-products, and other toxins, and begin breaking down some of the stored fat. Balanced nourishment with a low-fat, moderate-protein, complex-carbohydrate diet is recommended. Since alcoholics often have blood sugar problems, basic hypoglycemic principles should also be followed. These include avoiding sugars and refined foods such as soft drinks or candy, and eating every few hours. The basic diet consists of small meals and snacks of protein or complex carbohydrates including whole grains, pasta, potatoes, squashes, legumes, and other vegetables. Proteins such as soy products, eggs, fish, or poultry can also be added and small amounts of fruits and fruit juices may be tolerated. Since the primary aim is to maintain an alkaline diet, we should initially focus on vegetables and fruit. Of course, the Detox Diet can be used during the first two weeks of alcohol detoxification.

Water or herbal teas should be consumed throughout the day. Foods containing potentially damaging fats such as fast foods, lunch meats, chips, burgers, hot dogs, and ice cream should also be avoided, as they are all congesting and more acid-forming. Caffeine consumption and cigarette smoking are best minimized. Many people recovering from alcohol addiction consume large amounts of coffee and smoke intensely—an event seen clearly at AA meetings. I do not recommend this at all. Fortunately, there has been an increase in the number of nonsmoking AA meetings and nonsmoking recoverees.

During detoxification from alcohol, as with the other substances, supplemental nutrients are helpful. Herbal formulas, such as valerian root capsules, or prescription medicines can be used for sleep. Calcium and magnesium supplements taken at night may also aid sleep. L-glutamine, an amino acid that generates glutamic acid, can be used for energy. Glutamine is found naturally in liver, meats, dairy foods, and cabbage, and helps diminish the craving for alcohol and sugar. A dosage of 500–1,000 mg three times daily between or before meals is suggested, either in capsule or powdered form. Chromium may also help with sugar and alcohol cravings, at 200 mcg twice daily. Melatonin can also be used, and has had some good effects during detox for aiding sleep. A 3 mg tablet can be taken at bedtime.

A multiple vitamin with additional antioxidant nutrients is a good idea during detox from alcohol. Minerals such as zinc, iron, calcium, and magnesium should be taken to replace those lost during alcohol abuse. Higher levels of niacin, even up to 2 grams, along with 5–10 grams of vitamin C daily have been used with some success in alcohol withdrawal and detox. For basic support, vitamin C intake would be 500–1,000 mg taken four to six times daily.

Fiber helps bind toxins in the bowel and improve elimination. Choline and inositol, in doses of about 500 mg each three times daily, will improve fat digestion and utilization. Lemon water combined with a couple of teaspoons of olive oil and a quarter teaspoon or capsule of cayenne pepper will help detoxify the liver. You can decrease the oil absorption by taking fiber along with it, but olive oil alone is also thought to be nourishing to the liver and helpful in clearing chemical toxins. Cold-pressed olive oil is commonly used in many natural liver therapies. Milk thistle herb (*Silybum marianum* or *Silymarin*) offers protection and healing to the liver in detoxification. One or two capsules of goldenseal root powder twice daily is also helpful for toning and cleaning the liver. Parsley tea improves kidney elimination and cleanses the blood. The amino acid L-cysteine is another helpful detoxicant for the liver, blood, and colon.

Other nutrients and herbs can also be helpful. These include pancreatic digestive enzymes, taken after meals, and Brewer's yeast if tolerated, which supplies many B vitamins and minerals. The essential fatty acids help decrease the inflammatory prostaglandins. Gamma-linolenic acid from evening primrose or borage seed oil assists in the reduction of alcohol toxicity. White willow bark tablets can be used for pain, and valerian root, a natural and milder form of Valium, can be taken to decrease anxiety. Chamomile will help calm the digestive tract, as will licorice root.

Nutritional Support for Drinkers

The basic support plan for active drinkers resembles that which is used during complete alcohol detox. A generally balanced and nutritious diet will help minimize some of the potential problems from alcohol, although even the best diet and supplement program will not fully protect us from ethanol's toxic effects. When our liver is metabolizing alcohol, it is helpful to avoid fried foods, rancid or hydrogenated fats, and other drugs, all of which are hard on the liver. Thioctic (lipoic) acid may help protect the liver against some of the toxicity, as can milk thistle herb.

Alcohol users need more nutrients than most people to protect them from malnutrition. Obviously, basic multivitamins and antioxidant formulas are important. Part, or possibly most of, the toxic effects of alcohol may be caused by the production of free radicals. Higher-than-RDA levels of vitamins A, C, and E, beta-carotene, and the minerals selenium, zinc, manganese, and magnesium are suggested (see supplement table ahead for all dosages). Commonly deficient nutrients also need extra support. Thiamine, riboflavin, and niacin help circulation and blood cleansing and can reduce the effects of hangovers. I recommend folic acid in amounts more than twice the RDA; leafy greens and whole grains, both rich in this vitamin, should be added to the diet.

Water and other nonalcoholic liquids are needed to counteract the dehydrating effects of alcohol. Calcium is supportive, as is extra zinc, as its absorption is diminished and elimination is increased with alcohol use. This supplemental intake should be balanced out with copper. The essential fatty acids and gamma-linolenic acid from evening primrose oil or borage seed oil support normal fat metabolism and protect against inflammation caused by free radicals and prostaglandins (PGEs). Alcohol decreases the levels of the anti-inflammatory PGE_1, and these oils will begin to raise their levels again. Glutathione helps prevent fat buildup in the liver through its enzymatic activities, so the tripeptide glutathione (or L-cysteine, which forms glutathione) may be supplemented along with basic L-amino acids. Additional L-glutamine will enhance brain cell function.

Social Drinking

I recommend that social drinkers use a lighter version of this program, as they still need protection against alcohol's toxicity. A good diet is, of course, essential, plus vitamins B_1, B_2, and B_3, folic acid, and B_{12}. These, along with zinc (15-30 mg), magnesium (300-500 mg), and vitamin C (1,000 mg) should be taken with some food before drinking. In general, drinking should be limited to two drinks per day.

A number of things can help prevent drunkenness and hangover. Our alcohol blood level is affected by how much and how fast we drink and absorb. Drink slowly. If we drink fast on an empty stomach, absorption is immediate. Ideally, it is best to have some food in the stomach, or to limit consumption to one drink before eating. Food also prevents us from getting sick. I recommend low-salt complex carbohydrates such as bread, crackers, or vegetable sticks, because carbohydrates delay alcohol absorption. Fat-protein snacks such as milk or cheese will also decrease alcohol absorption, thus reducing drunkenness and hangovers. Some people even drink a little olive oil before parties to coat their stomachs before drinking. A few capsules of evening primrose oil will have a similar effect. Women seem to be more readily affected by alcohol than men, even when body weight is equal.

Once alcohol is ingested, it just takes time to clear it from the blood. With heavy drinking, extra coffee and exercise do not really help; however, with mild intoxication they can increase alertness. Definitely avoid other psychoactive drugs when drinking alcohol, including tranquilizers, narcotics, sedatives, antihistamines, and marijuana, all of which may increase alcohol's effect.

Alcohol blood levels have been studied in order to understand their varying effect. Tests are used to clarify degrees of safety while under the influence, versus more potentially dangerous drunkenness. Usually one or two drinks will leave people in the safe range, but more can create problems. Hangovers are caused both by the dehydrating effect of alcohol and by the toxic effects of the chemical congeners or sulfur compounds created during fermentation or added to the beverages. Allergies to some of the ingredients such as corn, wheat, barley, or yeast may intensify hangovers and withdrawal.

Alcohol Blood Level	Status
0.05 percent	"Cruising," feeling good, some positive effects
0.05–0.1	Beginning loss of balance, speech or emotions
0.08	Legally drunk
0.2	Passed out
0.3	Comatose, unresponsive

The best hangover remedy is to prevent them altogether by not overdrinking and taking supportive fluids and nutrients. Cream, coffee, oysters, chili peppers, and aspirin are common and occasionally helpful hangover remedies. Time is the only real remedy, however, along with rest and fluids. If alcohol intake has been excessive, drink two or three glasses of water before going to bed, along with some vitamin C and a B complex vitamin to clear alcohol from the blood. Repeat upon awakening. Emergen-C can also be used—it is a vitamin C powder with added vitamins and minerals, and is available at natural food stores. Evening primrose oil and flaxseed oil also help. A morning-after plan suggested by Dr. Stuart Berger includes 100 mg of thiamine, 100 mg of riboflavin, 50 mg of B_6, 250 mcg of B_{12}, 1,000 mg of vitamin C, and 50 mg of zinc.

Overall, we need to monitor our drinking and not let alcohol use turn into abuse and addiction. We need to pay special attention to children and teenagers and offer them education regarding alcohol and drugs and provide them with good role models in ourselves. Let us all live as examples of how we would like the world to be.

ALCOHOL NUTRIENT PROGRAMS			
	Support	Withdrawal	Detox/Recovery
Water	2 1/2–3 qt	3–4 qt	3 qt
Protein	60–80 g	50–70 g	75–100 g
Fats	30–50 g	30–50 g	50–65 g
Fiber	15–20 g	10–15 g	30–40 g
Vitamin A	10,000 IU	5,000 IU	10,000 IU
Beta-carotene	25,000 IU	20,000 IU	20,000 IU
Vitamin D	200 IU	400 IU	400 IU
Vitamin E	400–800 IU	400 IU	800 IU
Vitamin K	300 mcg	300 mcg	500 mcg
Thiamine (B_1)	100 mg	50–100 mg	150 mg

	Support	Withdrawal	Detox/Recovery
Riboflavin (B$_2$)	100 mg	50–100 mg	150 mg
Niacinamide (B$_3$)	50 mg	50 mg	50 mg
Niacin (B$_3$)	50–150 mg	100–1,000 mg	200–2,000 mg
Pantothenic acid (B$_5$)	250 mg	1,000 mg	500 mg
Pyridoxine (B$_6$)	100 mg	200 mg	100 mg
Pyridoxal-5-phosphate	50 mg	100 mg	50 mg
Cobalamin (B$_{12}$)	100 mcg	200 mcg	250 mcg
Folic acid	800–1,000 mcg	2,000 mcg	800 mcg
Biotin	300 mcg	500 mcg	500 mcg
Choline	500 mg	1,000 mg	1,500 mg
Inositol	500 mg	1,000 mg	1,500 mg
Vitamin C	2–4 g	5–25 g	5–10 g
Bioflavonoids	250 mg	500 mg	500 mg
Calcium*	850–1,000 mg	1,000–1,500 mg	1,000 mg
Chromium	500 mcg	500–1,000 mcg	300 mcg
Copper*	3 mg	3 mg	3–4 mg
Iodine	150 mcg	150 mcg	150 mcg
Iron*	15–30 mg	10–18 mg	20 mg
Magnesium*	500–800 mg	800–1,000 mg	600–800 mg
Manganese	5 mg	15 mg	10 mg
Molybdenum	300 mcg	300 mcg	300 mcg
Potassium*	300–500 mg	500 mg	300 mg
Selenium	300 mcg	150 mcg	200 mcg
Silicon	100 mg	50 mg	200 mg
Vanadium	150 mcg	150 mcg	150 mcg
Zinc*	45–75 mg	50–75 mg	50–100 mg
Flaxseed oil	1 teaspoon	2 teaspoons	2 teaspoons
Gamma-linolenic acid (40–60 mg/capsules)	3 capsules	3 capsules	6 capsules
L-amino acids	1,000–1,500 mg	1,500–3,000 mg	5,000–7,500 mg
L-glutamine	500–1,000 mg	1,500–3,000 mg	1,000–2,000 mg
Lipoic acid	100 mg	100 mg	200 mg
L-cysteine, or	250 mg	250 mg	250–500 mg
Glutathione	250 mg	500 mg	250 mg
Digestive enzymes	—	—	1–2 after meals
Goldenseal root	—	—	3 capsules
White willow bark (for pain)	1–2 tablets	4–6 tablets	2–4 tablets
Silymarin (milk thistle)	2–4 capsules	3 capsules	3–6 capsules

* Amounts may vary based on individual needs.

ALCHOHOL DETOX SUMMARY

1. If you have been drinking for a long time or drink large amounts, seek multi-level support. This gives you the best chance for a permanent change. Have professional support for this process.

2. If you consume more than 6 to 8 drinks daily, seriously consider inpatient help or a residential detox program.

3. A juice cleanse or the Detox Diet, often accompanied with light protein and amino acids, can be useful in the transition and detox process. Post-detox, whole foods with complex carbohydrates and adequate proteins can be nourishing.

4. Follow basic hypoglycemic guidelines—avoid sugars and sweetened foods, have some nourishment regularly (every 2 to 3 hours), maintain adequate protein intake.

5. Drink 6 to 8 glasses or more of water daily to help clear the liver and cleanse the body of toxins.

6. Include sufficient fiber to support proper bowel elimination.

7. Use nutritional supplements to support your body during detoxification from alcohol. Medically supervised intravenous (IV) nutrition of vitamins B and C along with minerals may also be useful.

8. Be sure to include antioxidant nutrients to help with detox—namely vitamins C and E, beta-carotene, zinc, and selenium.

9. Use specific herbs to cleanse and heal the liver and facilitate detoxification—these include milk thistle (silymarin), dandelion root, and others.

10. Consider acupuncture to treat physical cravings and withdrawal symptoms.

11. Get support that fits your own values—perhaps psychological counseling, family therapy, AA, or a religious or spiritual practice.

12. Avoid places and people which most trigger your drinking.

CHAPTER NINE

Nicotine Detoxification

◆

The cigarette is the world's most profitable globally distributed product. Why? Because nicotine is more addictive than either alcohol or cocaine.

Cigarette smoking, our primary method of using nicotine, is the single greatest cause of preventable disease and probably creates the most difficult addiction to deal with. The statistics are shocking: World-wide, 2.5 million people a year die of tobacco-related diseases. In the United States alone, cigarette smoking causes over 1,000 deaths per day and is responsible for about 25 percent of cancer deaths and 30 to 40 percent of coronary heart disease deaths. It also increases the incidence of atherosclerosis, strokes, and peripheral vascular disease. Diseases of the respiratory tract—colds, flus, acute bronchitis, pneumonia, chronic obstructive pulmonary diseases (COPD) such as emphysema and chronic bronchitis, and lung cancer—are all much more common in smokers. Infections and allergies are also prevalent in smokers, as is rapid aging of the body, especially facial skin, which results from the poor oxygenation of tissues and other associated chemical effects.

Smoking clearly decreases life expectancy for all age groups. One-pack-a-day smokers double their chance of death between ages 50 and 60, while two-packers triple theirs. (These statistics are reflected in the insurance rates smokers pay, which are twice that of non-smokers.) Smoking also affects the life expectancy of nonsmokers. Of all the commonly used drugs, nicotine has the least benefits and the greatest consequences.

In spite of these facts, some 650 billion cigarettes are sold yearly in the United States, creating an $18–25 billion megabusiness. The 650 billion count averages to about 4,000 cigarettes per year per person over the age of 18, although aggressive marketing and social pressure targets people even younger. The 1989 Surgeon General's Report stated that about half of all smokers begin before the age of fifteen. Recent estimates suggest that about 38 percent of the over-18 population in the United States smoke. Percentages of adult smokers are much higher in most European countries and parts of Asia. Billions of dollars are spent to treat the problems that afflict smokers and many more billions are lost due to decreased work and productivity.

Children getting hooked is the saddest part of the nicotine story. We must insist on more stringent laws to better regulate sales and advertising, along with better education to help curtail this problem.

Since most nicotine is ingested by smoking cigarettes, that is the focus of this chapter. Cigar and pipe smoking, chewing tobacco and snuff also pose health risks, but far fewer than with cigarettes. Tobacco comes from a large-leafed nightshade, or Solanaceae, plant. It is one of only a few plants that contain the psychoactive alkaloid nicotine. Tobacco causes joint pain in some people, which correlates with the theory that arthritis is in part due to a nightshade allergy.

The highly addictive nature of nicotine is revealed by the fact that many strong-minded and strong-willed people cannot stop smoking, even if they are otherwise health conscious. Over 80 percent of smokers say that they want to stop. In my years working in hospitals, I saw lung cancer and emphysema patients smoking between ventilator treatments and patients with tubes in their necks from tracheostomies putting cigarettes into the tubes to inhale.

Nicotine Effects and Benefits (yes, there are a few)

Many people find smoking to be relaxing, but this may be related to the way it calms hyperactive withdrawal symptoms. People do experience increased mental stimulation and improved hand-to-eye coordination as a result of nicotine's vascular-neurological stimulation, but the effects do not last.

The "up" feeling that smoking produces is probably correlated with increased blood pressure and heart rate, as well as the production of fatty acids, steroids, hormones, and neurotransmitters. Nicotine mimics acetylcholine, which improves alertness, memory, and learning capacity. Stimulation of norepinephrine and endorphins by nicotine may help balance moods and increase energy. The liver's increased glycogen release gives a satisfying lift to the blood sugar.

Dr. Tom Ferguson's book, *The Smoker's Book of Health*, cites how hundreds of smokers said they felt better able to deal with stress and to relax with nicotine. Smoking helped control their moods, improved concentration and energy levels (especially with fatigue), and reduced withdrawal symptoms. Social comfort, work breaks, reduced pain and anxiety, increased pleasure, and less boredom were also noted.

Smoking also reduces one's appetite and taste for food, a benefit for the weight conscious. In fact, the average smoker weighs six to eight pounds less than the nonsmoker. In *Life Extension*, Sandy Shaw and Durk Pearson note that nicotine seems to reduce distraction by outside stimuli in people working in highly stimulating environments—that is, it desensitizes people.

Nicotine is a mild central nervous system stimulant and a strong cardiovascular system stimulant. It constricts blood vessels, increasing blood pressure and stimulating the heart, and raises blood fat levels. In its liquid form, nicotine is a powerful poison—the injection of even one drop would be deadly. Interestingly, it is the nicotine, not the smoke, that causes people to continue smoking cigarettes, yet it is the smoking itself that causes so many of the health problems.

The initial irritating effects of nicotine easily progress to chronic irritations, yet these are outweighed by the physiological and psychological dependence. People addicted to heroine and other powerful drugs have commonly cited nicotine as the hardest drug to kick. The American Psychiatric Association has described smoking as an "organic mental disorder." Their statistics suggest that around 50 percent of people cannot stop smoking when they try to and that, of the people who do stop, about 75 percent of them begin again within one year.

Cigarette smoke is a combination of lethal gases (carbon monoxide, hydrogen cyanide, and nitrogen and sulfur oxides) and tars (which contain an estimated 4,000 chemicals). Some of the chemical agents are introduced by the actual manufacturing processes. Tobacco has been smoked for centuries, and it has until recently been naturally grown and dried. It appears that in the last century, as chemicals have been added, the negative effects of smoking have skyrocketed. Research suggests that natural tobacco poses much less cancer and cardiovascular disease risk than processed tobacco.

What are the Risks of Smoking?

Dangers in modern tobacco products include pesticides used during cultivation and chemicals added to the tobacco to make it burn better or taste different. Chemicals added to the leaves and papers to enhance burning are the major cause of fire death in this country, as those cigarettes continue to burn after they have been put down. Forced burning also makes people smoke more of each cigarette in order to keep up with it. Sugar curing and rapid flue drying are also associated with increased toxicity. Kerosene heat drying contaminates the tobacco with yet another toxic hydrocarbon.

Using a natural tobacco may reduce smoking risks; if a cigarette does not go out when left alone, it has been chemically treated.

Other toxic contaminants in cigarettes include cadmium (which affects the kidneys, arteries, and blood pressure), lead, arsenic, cyanide, and nickel. Dioxin, the most toxic pesticide chemical known, has been found in cigarettes, as has acetonitrile, another pesticide. The nitrogen gases from cigarettes generate carcinogenic nitrosamines in body tissues. The tars in smoke contain polynuclear aromatic hydrocarbons (PAH), carcinogenic materials that bind with cellular DNA to cause damage. Antioxidant therapy, particularly with vitamin C, helps protect against both PAH and nitrosamines. Extra C blocks the irritating effects of smoke and replaces what is lost due to reduced absorption (blood levels of ascorbic acid average about 30–40 percent lower in smokers than in nonsmokers).

Radioactive materials are also found in cigarette smoke, polonium being the most common. Some authorities believe that cigarettes are our greatest source of radiation, which is a strong aging factor. A smoker of one and a half packs per day may be exposed to radiation levels equal to 300 chest x-rays yearly. Acetaldehyde, a chemical released during smoking, also causes aging (especially of the skin) as it affects the cross-linking bonds that hold our tissues together.

There are different levels of addiction. Least addicted are those who smoke socially—only at parties with friends—and usually only during certain times of the day or week. Next are those who smoke in response to stress, mainly at work, and who may stop and start periodically. These two types usually find it easier to cut down or stop. Those of us who are all-day-long smokers have a strong physical and psychological addiction. Going more than an hour without nicotine brings on withdrawal symptoms such as irritability, anxiety, or headache. Often, the psychological factors are more intense than the physical ones. Consuming two or more packs a day indicates a strong addiction; medical and psychological support will likely be necessary to quit successfully. Specialized smoking-cessation programs are often useful.

Contrary to current marketing hype about low-tar, low-nicotine cigarettes, there are no safe smoking options. Some of the newer "lights" may be even worse than regular cigarettes as users inhale more deeply and smoke more frequently in order to satisfy nicotine needs. More carbon monoxide, hydrogen cyanide, and nitrogen gases are consumed with many of these low-nicotine cigarettes, and this can increase the oxygen deficit, heart disease, and lung damage associated with smoking. What smokers really need are high-nicotine, low-tar cigarettes, so that they will smoke less for the same amount of nicotine. Even better would be a way to get nicotine to the blood without smoke at all. Nicotine gum works well, and nicotine skin patches are now used in smoking-cessation programs. Nicotine nasal sprays have just been released, and soon there may be capsules or tablets to satisfy the craving. All of these options will still be moderately hazardous to our health, but much less so than smoking. They will also get rid of the primary and secondary risks due to smoke and smoke-born chemicals.

Although about a third of adult men and women in the United States smoke, over one million of the over 50 million smokers in the United States stop smoking each year; when we do this, we immediately begin to lower our potential for disease.

Cigarette smoking puts us at risk through three primary degenerative-disease producing effects: 1) irritation and inflammation; 2) free-radical generation; and 3) allergy-addiction. Respiratory and cardiovascular diseases are the greatest and deadliest long-term consequences of smoking.

PROBLEMS ASSOCIATED WITH SMOKING

Cough	Allergies	Cancers
Hoarseness	Rhinitis/sinusitis	Lung
Headaches	Lowered immunity	Mouth and Tongue
Anxiety	Other infections	Larynx
Fatigue	Blood disorders	Esophagus
Leg pains	Nutrient deficiencies	Bladder
Cold hands and feet	Acute bronchitis	Cervix
Memory loss	Chronic bronchitis	Pancreas
Senility	Emphysema	Kidney
Alzheimer's disease	Increased cholesterol	Surgical complications
Rapid skin aging	Atherosclerosis	Increased pregnancy risks
Teeth and finger stains	Hypertension	Increased infant mortality
Periodontal disease	Angina Pectoris	Burns from fires
Low libido	Circulation insufficiency	Increased caffeine use
Impotence	Heart and artery disease	Increased alcohol use
Heartburn	Heart attacks and strokes	More job and home changes
Peptic ulcers	Varicose veins	Higher insurance and
Hiatal hernia	Osteoporosis	medical fees

- **Cardiovascular disease (CVD),** or the process of artherosclerosis, from the inflammatory effects and cholesterol-increasing effects of nicotine on the circulatory system.
- CVD from carbon monoxide in inhaled smoke which reduces the delivery of oxygen to our cells.
- Reduced oxygen levels cause our body to produce more red blood cells (polycythemia).
- CVD is primarily responsible for the **decreased life expectancy** associated with smoking, even more so than with lung cancer which usually only arises after 20–30 years of use, while circulatory effects start immediately.
- The three primary contributors to CVD are *smoking, hypertension,* and *high cholesterol,* and smoking increases the incidence of the latter two.
- Nicotine also lowers the level of the protective HDL cholesterol.
- Decreased circulation and increased peripheral vascular resistance cause the heart to work harder with every beat and contributes to **elevated blood pressure.**
- Increased platelet aggregation leads to **strokes and heart attacks.** Smokers are three times more likely than nonsmokers to suffer **heart attacks,** mostly of the artery-spasm type. The pre-heart-attack propensity to **angina pectoris** is also higher. Nicotine (and other agents in smoke) increase the incidence of **arrhythmias** (irregular heartbeat).
- **Cerebral aneurysm** (ballooning of the artery wall) may also be fatal.
- **Peripheral vascular disease** (disease of the arteries in the extremities) may manifest as **intermittent claudication** (pain in the legs when walking), as the poor circulation caused by atherosclerosis and vasoconstriction reduces oxygen delivery to the muscles.
- **Buerger's disease** is an arterial disease that may be caused by a hypersensitivity or allergy to tobacco. The inflammation and scarring of the arteries in the arms and legs may even lead to amputation.
- Chronic inhalation of tobacco smoke eventually **destroys lung tissues** through a process of irritation, inflammation, and scarring.
- A higher than average incidence of **respiratory infections,** including colds and flus, bronchitis and sinusitis. Cigarette smoke causes temporary paralysis of the cilia (fine hairs on the mucous linings which protect the deeper tissues from microorganisms and other foreign materials). The thinning and drying of the mucus itself dries and irritates the bronchial tubes.
- **Chronic bronchitis,** one form of **chronic obstructive pulmonary disease (COPD),** results from long-term irritation, loss of mucus protection, and recurrent infection with a subsequent **loss of lung capacity** and function. This limitation in respiratory function occurs very near the onset of smoking. When smoking is stopped, much of the

function returns, unless there is lung tissue scarring which is irreversible.

- Smoking generally decreases lung capacity and endurance and with it, the desire or ability to exercise. **Emphysema,** another form of COPD, results from progressive scarring and loss of lung elasticity.

- Smokers are from five to ten times more likely to contract **lung cancer** than nonsmokers. These rates are even further increased with occupational exposure to agents such as asbestos, coal, textiles, and other chemicals. With regular alcohol use, smokers have greater than fifteen times the risk of lung cancer than nonsmokers.

- Many other cancer rates are also higher for smokers, particularly for alcohol-drinking smokers who are exposed to other carcinogenic chemicals.

- **Allergy-addiction symptoms** may appear when smoking is first begun and then decrease with continued smoking.

- Increased atherosclerosis and subsequent decrease in blood circulation to the brain lead to **memory loss** and thinking problems, as well as early dementia. Recent research shows that smokers have four times greater the risk of **Alzheimer's disease.**

- Poor oxygen delivery to the skin and general dehydration of the tissues caused by smoking **ages the skin** and increases the number of deep wrinkles.

- Worldwide reports show how smoking affects **sexuality** and **reproduction.** In **men,** smoking has been shown to **lower sperm counts and reproductive ability.** Smoking may also cause genetic mutation, as there appears to be a slightly higher incidence of congenital malformations in the offspring of men who smoke.

- In **women** who smoke, there are clearly more **miscarriages** and **babies with lower birth weights.**

- Smoking also increases the incidence of **stillbirths, congenital malformations,** and **early infant deaths.**

- Smoking around newborns and infants increases their susceptibility to many diseases, particularly **colds, ear infections, bronchitis,** and **pneumonia.**

- Women are at risk for all of the problems described above, but are particularly vulnerable if they are using birth control pills. For example, women who smoke and use the pill are 25 times more likely to suffer from **heart attacks** than women who do neither.

- Although **snuff** and **chewing tobacco** are less toxic, chronic use of the nicotine affects the circulatory system. There are currently over 10 million chewers addicted to nicotine; even though they are not exposed to smoke, they still have the negative cardiovascular effects and a higher incidence of mouth, tongue, and throat cancers than smokers. The smoke from **cigars** and **pipes** is not usually inhaled, so less nicotine and tars are absorbed with their use, although local irritation is possible.

- Smoking reduces appetite and taste for food, thus **interfering with good nutrition.**
- Increased risk of **osteoporosis** due to poor calcium utilization.
- Increased incidence of **heartburn, hiatal hernia, and peptic ulcers.**

HIGH RISK SMOKERS

Pregnant women	Obese people
Nursing mothers	Very thin people
Diabetics	Alcoholics or alcohol abusers
Women using birth control pills	People with existing smoker's disease
Family history of heart disease	People who work with toxic chemicals
Hypertensives	People having surgery
People with high cholesterol	Ulcer patients
Heavy smokers	Type A personalities

What About Secondary Smoke?

Secondary smoke has become a human rights issue in the last decade as people feel that it is a violation of their right to breathe clean air. Secondhand smoke is potentially more dangerous than mainstream smoke because it is not filtered. Of the 16 or so poisons that arise from burning cigarettes, most are known carcinogens. Much of the ammonia, formaldehyde, acetaldehyde, formic acid, phenol, hydrogen sulfide, acetonitrile, and methyl chloride is filtered through the cigarette filters and is more concentrated in the smoke that wafts into the air. This is the smoke that passive, involuntary smokers inhale. Carbon monoxide levels in secondhand smokers is more than 50 percent higher than that of those not exposed and often even exceeds that of light firsthand smokers.

A review of more than 2,000 studies regarding secondhand smoke suggest that it increases the incidence of most of the diseases associated with smoking. Children of smokers have increased incidence of respiratory infections, ear infections, and lower lung function than children of nonsmokers. Secondhand smoke increases the risk of COPD, heart disease, and lung cancer. In fact, an estimated 3,000 cases of lung cancers a year are caused by secondhand smoking. It has been found that nonsmoking wives of male smokers have life expectancies that are four years shorter than those of nonsmoking wives of nonsmokers.

How Do We Detoxify from Nicotine?

A good air filter is an important preventative measure and can be very effective in removing toxins from the air; a basic multiple vitamin-mineral and antioxidant formula will help protect us internally. The daily program should include at least:

SMOKER'S SIMPLE NUTRIENT PLAN	
Vitamin C	1,000–2,000 mg
Beta-carotene*	15,000–25,000 IU
Vitamin A	5,000–10,000 IU
Zinc	15–30 mg
Selenium	200 mcg
Vitamin E	400 IU

* Note: Even though beta-carotene did not fair well in recent studies for smoker's when used solely, I believe its action within a complete antioxidant formula is still warranted based on a number of other positive studies.

Dietary Recommendations

No support program for smokers will be as effective as ceasing to smoke completely and working to regain lost health. A wholesome diet and nutritional supplements can help protect us from some of the effects of smoking; however, even the best program cannot offer immunity. There is a tendency for poor dietary habits to accompany the destructive smoking habit. Many smokers tend to eat more meats, fatty, fried, and refined foods than nonsmokers, although I have seen smoking vegetarians, smoking exercise fanatics, and smoking health enthusiasts.

This plan, with adequate fruits, vegetables, and whole grains, will help to replenish the protective antioxidant nutrients such as beta-carotene, vitamins A, C, and E, and selenium. In addition, raw seeds and nuts, legumes, sprouts, and other proteins should be consumed. Water is essential to balance out the drying effects of smoking. Caffeine also increases the need for water, as it is dehydrating. A daily intake of two to three quarts of liquid is suggested, depending on how many high-water-content fruits, vegetables, salads, and soups are consumed.

Since smoking usually generates an acidic condition in the body, I recommend the Detox Diet. A high-fiber diet helps detoxification by maintaining bowel function.

The nutritional strategy for smokers is to increase the intake of wholesome foods—fruits, vegetables, and whole grains—and to decrease the intake of fats, cured or pickled products, food additives, and alcohol. The increased blood and tissue alkalinity that results from this diet helps reduce the craving for and interest in smoking, as shown by studies and my patients' reports.

An alkaline diet is not necessarily needed over an entire lifetime, although generally, it is preferable to an acid diet. During cigarette withdrawal, a vegetarian or raw food diet may sufficiently reduce nicotine craving, and can be used for three to six weeks to aid in the detoxification process. Fasting has also been employed by some smokers to help eliminate their habit. It is a means of rapid transition, but is also somewhat intense. A juice fast under medical supervision might best be used with the very determined person or with the overweight or hypertensive smoker.

STOP SMOKING DIET			
Increase Alkaline Foods		**Reduce Acid Foods**	
fruits	figs	meats	beef
vegetables	raisins	sugar	chicken
greens	carrots	wheat	eggs
lima beans	celery	bread	milk
millet	almonds	baked goods	cheese

Several weeks of the Detox Diet (p. 35) can be very effective at clearing the desire, habit, and chemicals from the body. Over a longer time, a vegetarian diet high in chlorophyllic (green) vegetables and sprouts, grains, fruits, and liquids such as water, juices, soups, and herbal teas is preferable. The raw foods diet is similar, but includes more seeds and nuts. Eating raw, unsalted sunflower seeds (or carrot or celery sticks) can help replace that hand-to-mouth habit we reinforce when we smoke. How-ever, we must be careful not to replace nicotine addiction with new food addictions.

The diet for detoxification is low in fat and high in fiber, helping to keep energy levels high and the gut cleansed. Raw and vegetarian foods help with both. The diet includes several salads of leafy greens daily, and some fruit, vegetable, nut, or seed snacks. Some of the high-protein algae such as spirulina, blue-green algae, or chlorella also help during withdrawal and detox.

Supplements

To support body alkalinization during smoking cessation, I recommend sodium or potassium bicarbonate tablets, taking one during each period of craving up to a total of five or six tablets daily. A general "multiple" vitamin with additional antioxidant nutrients is an important part of the smoker's program (please see page 105 for all dosages). The antioxidants help reduce the toxicity of smoke in primary and secondary smokers and also help lessen free-radical irritation during the detox period. Vitamin E helps stabilize cell membranes, protecting them and the tissue membranes from free-radical and chemical irritations. Selenium, as sodium selenite or selenomethionine, supports vitamin E and also reduces cancer potential. Selenium also lessens sensitivity to cadmium. Vitamin A reduces cancer risk and supports tissue health; beta-carotene may protect against lung cancer when used with other antioxidants. Therefore, smokers need regular vitamin C intake to help neutralize the toxins and compensate for reduced absorption. (Note: Both vitamin C and niacin are mild acids, which may increase ulcer risk and nicotine craving in smokers. If C or niacin are used in higher amounts, extra alkaline salts such as the bicarbonates or calcium-magnesium ascorbates may be used.) Extra zinc, 30–60 mg a day, like vitamin A, helps protect the tissue and mucous membranes and reduces cadmium toxicity and absorption. If higher levels of zinc (over 60 mg daily) are taken, supplement with 3–4 mg copper.

We need the support of the B vitamins, particularly thiamine (B_1), pyridoxine (B_6), and cobalamin (B_{12}). B_{12} is thought to help decrease the cellular damage caused by tars and nicotine. Niacin (B_3) helps open up constricted circulation. It also lowers cholesterol, which may reduce the risk of atherosclerosis. Pantothenic acid (B_5) may reduce skin aging and the effects of stress. Folic acid should be taken in higher amounts. Coenzyme Q_{10} can be helpful, and extra choline supports the brain and memory. Magnesium and molybdenum are also needed in higher amounts than usual.

L-cysteine (along with thiamine and vitamin C) protects the lungs from acetaldehyde generated by smoking, and helps reduce smoker's cough. Glutathione, formed from L-cysteine, is part of the protective antioxidant enzyme system. Heavy smokers might use 250–500 mg of glutathione, up to 1,500 mg (usually 500–750 mg) of L-cysteine, with 5–6 g of vitamin C, 150 mg thiamine, and the total B vitamins and a balanced amino acid formula daily.

To prevent obesity during and following smoking cessation, it is very important to be aware of our eating habits. Since smoking reduces appetites and increases metabolism, it is natural to want to eat more when not smoking. Replace smoking with exercise or new activities. Research has shown that smokers crave and eat less sweets than nonsmokers; however, this changes with smoking cessation as the taste buds come alive again. Over half of ex-smokers will gain weight when they stop smoking, and this is even more common in the heavier-use smokers. If weight gain is undesirable (many smokers are underweight and should gain weight), a weight-control diet should be instituted as smoking is stopped. The alkaline, high-fiber, low-fat diet is helpful in maintaining weight. Another amino acid, L-phenylalanine, can help reduce the appetite if taken before meals in amounts of 250–500 mg. However, its mild tendency to raise blood pressure should be taken into consideration. (This may be countered by the tendency of the blood pressure to drop somewhat with smoking cessation.) More choline may improve fat utilization and maintain weight, as may the amino acid L-carnitine. Regular exercise and plenty of fresh air are also part of the plan.

The level of nicotine addiction is based upon daily amounts and total number of years smoking, and will determine the ease of cessation. If you light up first thing in the morning or if you smoke more than two packs a day, it may be harder for you to stop than for lighter smokers.

Stop-Smoking Plans

There are many different cessation plans. The best way is just to make a firm decision and go cold turkey—there is no back and forth, no doubt; the decision is made. The success rate for those who make this bold move is much better than for those who use other methods. They do not need tapes, counselors, or group support; they count on themselves. Those who depend on others to stop smoking have more relapses.

Withdrawal is not easy. The first three days to a week can be very difficult; for some people, the struggle may last for months. Usually, the first 12–24 hours are the peak of withdrawal, when symptoms may appear and when cigarette craving is almost omnipresent. During withdrawal, I suggest taking one gram of vitamin C (as a mineral ascorbate to reduce acidity) every one or two hours. This may help reduce nicotine cravings.

If you just cannot give up nicotine, there are other ways to get rid of cigarettes. Though not ideal, they are at least one step better than smoking. Nicorette, a nicotine gum, is now available without prescription and can be a very useful transitional tool; more recently, nicotine patches in varying strengths are also being used. Both of these methods support nicotine addiction without harmful smoke chemicals. They reduce withdrawal symptoms, and research suggests a better long-term quitting percentage for those using nicotine gum and patches. These are, however, temporary aids. These substances may cause nausea, lightheadedness, hiccups, and muscle tension or jaw aches from chewing. They do, however, immediately help one to stop smoking, as most of the nicotine craving is satisfied. The smoking response must still be addressed, and the former smoker should be off the gum or patches within a couple of months, or sometimes longer. (Patches may even need to be used for a year to be successful.) Research suggests that people with ulcers or cardiovascular disease should avoid these methods, as should pregnant women. "Smokeless" cigarettes can be used for withdrawal and transition as well.

If none of these methods are successful for you, there are many self-help suggestions for cutting down. Working to smoke fewer cigarettes daily is a common practice, but generally ten per day is needed to satisfy the nicotine habit. You might also try taking fewer puffs per cigarette or smoking just the first half of each, where the least amounts of tars and chemicals are concentrated. Filters and cigarette holders decrease the amount of toxic elements inhaled. There are also devices that place tiny holes in cigarette filters to allow dilution of smoke with outside air. You might also try changing brands to lower-tar, higher-nicotine cigarettes, or using brands you do not like. For anyone who smokes, I suggest avoiding chemically-treated cigarettes and using natural, untreated tobacco and untreated paper.

Compose a plan and schedule of cessation dates and stages of nonsmoking before quitting, and document your reasons for doing so. Pick a low-stress time to stop, such as during vacation or just after sick leave from work or school. New Year's Day, your birthday, or national stop smoking days are other good choices. Keep notes of your process and feelings. Get to know yourself better through this process; many smokers release a lot of energy and excitement as they quit, so use this to construct new and better habits in all areas of your life.

When you quit, make a commitment. If you have trouble doing this, find someone with lung cancer or emphysema to talk with. Know your cigarette triggers and work to defuse them. Get rid of ashtrays, clean your teeth and your home, and make your life a nonsmoking zone. Take extra special care of yourself with good foods, pure drinking water, hot baths or showers, exercise, and massage. Reward yourself with a trip to the mountains, an afternoon off at the movies, a day at a spa or beauty salon. Get your mind off yourself by getting involved with others; try volunteer work; coach a softball team; organize a fund-raiser for your community. Learn a new language or musical instrument; try gardening or a new sport.

SUGGESTIONS FOR SMOKING CESSATION

- Cut down on other addictive substances, such as caffeine, sugar, and alcohol, all of which can increase the desire to smoke.

- Get another smoker to stop with you or, even better, get an ex-smoker to support you while you stop.

- Tell empathetic friends or family and ask for their support—that is, go public with your plan to stop.

- Stay busy to prevent boredom and to keep your mind off smoking.

- Exercise regularly to decrease withdrawal, increase motivation, and increase relaxation. Include your favorite aerobic sport and try to do it outdoors.

- If you are not an exerciser, consider taking yoga, swimming, or low-impact aerobics.

- Create rewards for being successful and implement them daily.

- Get plenty of rest.

- Drink fluids and use water for therapy by taking showers, baths, saunas, or hot tubs, or by going swimming.

- Change daily patterns to avoid stimulating old smoking conditioning. This may include staying away from bars, alcohol, and coffee, avoiding friends who smoke, not receiving or making phone calls at specific locations in which you usually smoked, and getting up and doing something right after a meal.

- Learn and practice relaxation and breathing techniques.

- Practice visualization.

- Keep a positive attitude toward health and life.

- Get health treatments, such as massage or teeth cleaning to remove cigarette stains.

- Find temporary oral substitutes to deal with psychological ties to smoking. Oral fixation substitutes could include munchies such as vegetable sticks (carrot, celery, zucchini), apples, nuts, popcorn, sunflower seeds (unsalted) in shells, sugarless hard candies or nonedible substitutes such as gum; or chewing or sucking on ice cubes, toothpicks, licorice sticks, or drinking straws.

- If cravings arise, find ways to deal with them: Take a short break, a walk, a shower, drink tea, or do things with your hands, such as sketching or doodling, working a cross-word puzzle, or making a shopping list. Breathe and relax, and be thankful you are not smoking.

It is crucial for people who stop smoking to become highly skilled at handling stress. Most people who start smoking again do so when they are under increased stress. Relaxation tapes, classes, and counseling can help. Stress-reduction plans and exercises—both mental and physical—are also helpful. Use your own support system at these times. These plans for exercise and stress management are best initiated before smoking cessation, so the necessary tools will already be in place. Also, regular exercise and relaxation may reinforce the need to cut down or quit. In fact, regular exercise offers many of the same feelings smokers get from nicotine such as an "up" feeling, confidence, and a greater ability to relax and concentrate.

It is important to maintain a positive attitude and use affirmations such as "I am not a smoker" or "stopping smoking is a great benefit to my health." Or try this, "I am not a cigarette or an ashtray. I am not supporting the greedy cigarette industry; they don't pay my health insurance." Write them down and post them in specific areas as reminders. Many ex-smokers use negative imagery to stay away from cigarettes. They think of lung damage, heart disease, wrinkled skin, or limited activity whenever they feel the urge to smoke. If we visualize these negative images when we take a deep breath and hold it, the negative feedback we feel while oxygen levels are decreasing and carbon dioxide levels are rising will help us stay off cigarettes. We should remind ourselves that we are grappling with a substance more addicting than heroin, scientifically designed to keep us involved as paying customers—then banish it. Even more important is visualizing the positive benefits, such as the new ability to taste and smell, better digestion, improved respiratory and circulatory functions, and the chance for a longer and healthier life. Increasing the love we have for ourselves as nonsmokers and continuing to see ourselves as nonsmokers are key. Every day we are not smoking, we are making progress toward improved health.

STOP SMOKING BREW

Lemon grass	3 parts	Red clover leaf	2 parts	Mullein leaf	2 parts
Dandelion root	3 parts	Alfalfa	2 parts	Valerian root	1 part
Raspberry leaf	2 parts	Peppermint	2 parts	Catnip	1 part

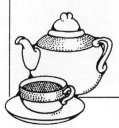

Simmer dandelion and valerian in water for 10 minutes, then pour into a pot containing other herbs and steep for 15 minutes. Use about 1 teaspoon of root and 1 tablespoon of leaves and flowers per cup of water. Drink one cup several times daily or as needed for cravings.

Smoking the herbs themselves has been used to replace cigarettes temporarily or to treat bronchopulmonary problems. Mullein leaf is probably the most commonly used. Coltsfoot, yerba santa, sarsaparilla, and rosemary have also been smoked. Lobelia leaf, called "Indian tobacco," has been employed as a cigarette substitute as it acts and tastes a bit like tobacco. In China, other herbs are smoked to treat asthma and other respiratory problems. Datura leaf is sometimes used, but can be slightly toxic. Ginseng leaf and other herbal cigarettes have been available. Smoking mugwort or catnip may help in relaxation; damiana is thought to have aphrodisiac properties; peppermint added to other blends gives a cool, menthol taste and licorice adds a sweet flavor. Chewing licorice sticks replaces the oral habit and settles the system. Chewing calamus root is a nicotine version of Antabuse. Garlic (taken orally, not smoked) is also helpful during the tobacco detox period.

A program that combines other supportive therapies, including acupuncture, counseling, hypnosis and massage, with diet and supplements works wonderfully, but can be time consuming and costly. Consider adding one of these forms of support to your plan. There are a number of good smoking cessation programs available in most cities and often the cost commitment and group support add extra incentive. However, I suggest avoiding rapid smoking plans that make you sicker to get well, as the excessive nicotine you will ingest can be toxic. A desire to stop and the willpower to continue pursuing a nonsmoking lifestyle is at the heart of all successful programs.

The nutrient levels in the following table can be spread out in several portions throughout the day. Vitamin C can be used even more frequently. The dosages range from smoker's support (low) to complete nicotine withdrawal (high), with the three to six weeks of initial detoxification requiring a mid-range amount.

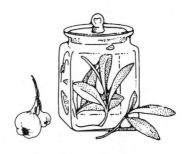

NICOTINE NUTRIENT PROGRAM

Water	2–3 qt	Copper	2–4 mg
Fat (low)	30–50 g	Iodine	150–250 mcg
Fiber	15–45 g	Iron*	women—20–30 mg
Vitamin A	10,000–15,000 IU		men—10–15 mg
Beta-carotene	20,000–40,000 IU	Magnesium	500–1,000 mg
Vitamin D	200–400 IU	Manganese	5–10 mg
Vitamin E	400–800 IU	Molybdenum	300–600 mcg
Vitamin K	100–300 mcg	Potassium	200–500 mg
Thiamine (B$_1$)	100–200 mg	Selenium	200–400 mcg
Riboflavin (B$_2$)	50–100 mg	Silicon	50–150 mg
Niacinamide (B$_3$)	50–100 mg	Vanadium	150–300 mcg
Niacin (B$_3$)	100–1,000 mg	Zinc	30–75 mg
Pantothenic acid (B$_5$)	250–1,000 mg	Coenzyme Q$_{10}$	50-100 mg
Pyridoxine (B$_6$)	50–150 mg	L-amino acids	1,000–2,000 mg
Pyridoxal-5-phosphate	25–75 mg	L-cysteine or	500–1,500 mg
Cobalamin (B$_{12}$)	200–1,000 mcg	Glutathione	250–500 mg
Folic acid	800–2,000 mcg	Essential fatty acids	4–6 capsules
Biotin	200–500 mcg	or Flaxseed oil	2–3 teaspoons
Choline	500–1,000 mg		
PABA	500–1,500 mg	**For withdrawal and detox:**	
Vitamin C	3–12 g	Garlic	3–6 capsules
Bioflavonoids	250–750 mg	Valerian root	4–6 capsules
Calcium	850–1,250 mg	Lobelia leaf	1–2 capsules
Chromium	200–500 mcg	Carrot sticks	10–20

* levels depend on body needs and blood loss

NICOTINE DETOX SUMMARY

1. Eat an alkaline diet of fruits, vegetables and whole grains. Follow the Detox Diet, or try a vegetarian or raw foods diet during detox. Reduce acid foods and potential carcinogens, such as fats, food additives, and alcohol.

2. Drink 2 to 3 quarts of pure water a day.

3. Keep fiber intake high to support detoxification and colon function.

4. Maintain vitamin levels through supplementation (see previous page). If cravings are strong, take 1 gram of vitamin C every 1 to 2 hours.

5. Also, take sodium or potassium bicarbonate tablets to alkalinize your body—one for each occasion of craving, but not more than 6 daily.

6. Use herbal supplements, including herbal stop-smoking brews.

7. Exercise, especially in the fresh air, to oxygenate your body.

8. If you are having real difficulty stopping, consider the use of nicotine patches or gum to help your transition.

9. Use acupuncture or hypnosis to motivate you to stop and/or to support you in withdrawal and detox.

10. Ease detox with relaxing therapies—hot baths or showers, saunas or hot tubs, swimming, massage.

11. Practice relaxation and deep breathing.

12. Build a method of support into your plan, including friends, family, and counseling. Stay busy and know that you are taking care of yourself, especially for the future.

13. Find oral substitutes for smoking. Change daily patterns to avoid smoking stimuli.

CHAPTER TEN

Fasting and Juice Cleansing

Fasting is the single greatest natural healing therapy I know. It is nature's ancient, universal remedy for many problems, used instinctively by animals when ill and by earlier cultures for healing and spiritual purification. When I first discovered fasting over 20 years ago, I felt as if it had saved my life. My stagnant energies began flowing, my allergies, aches, and pains disappeared, and I became more creative and vitally alive. I still find fasting both a useful personal tool and an important therapy for many medical and life problems.

Most of the conditions for which I recommend fasting are ones that result from excess nutrition rather than undernourishment. Dietary abuses generate many chronic degenerative diseases such as atherosclerosis, hypertension, heart disease, allergies, diabetes, cancer, and substance abuse which undermine our health and precede the breakdown of the body. I believe that fasting is not only therapeutic but, more importantly, acts as a preventative for many conditions. It often becomes the catalyst for shifting from unhealthy or abusive habits to a more healthful lifestyle in general.

As I use the term here, fasting refers to the avoidance of solid food and the intake of liquids only. True fasting would be the total avoidance of anything by mouth. The most stringent form of fasting allows drinking water exclusively; more liberal fasting includes the juices of fresh fruit and vegetables as well as herbal teas. All of these methods generate a high degree of detoxification—eliminating toxins from the body. Individual experiences with fasting depend upon the overall condition of our body, mind, and attitude. Detoxification can be intense and may either temporarily increase sickness or be immediately helpful and uplifting.

Juice fasting is commonly used as an effective cleansing plan. Fresh juices are easily assimilated and require minimum digestion, while still supplying many nutrients and stimulating our body to clear wastes. It is also safer than water fasting as it supports the body nutritionally while cleansing and hence maintains bodily energy levels, producing better detoxification and a quicker recovery.

I believe that fasting is the "missing link" in the Western diet. Most people overeat, eat too often, and eat a high-protein, high-fat, acid-congesting diet more consistently than is necessary. If we regularly eat a balanced, well-combined, more "alkalinizing" diet we will have less need for fasting and toning plans (although both are still highly beneficial, performed at intervals throughout the year).

Detoxification is a time when we allow our cells and organs to breathe and restore themselves. However, we do not necessarily need to fast to experience some cleansing. Even minor dietary shifts will initiate and promote better detox function, including an increase in fluids, more raw foods, and fewer congesting foods. For example, a vegetarian or macrobiotic diet will be very cleansing and purifying. The general process of detoxification is discussed thoroughly in Chapter 2: General Detoxification; here we focus on fluid fasting's history, benefits, and therapeutic use.

Fasting is a time-proven remedy, with human origins going back many thousands of years. Voluntary abstinence from food has been a tradition in most religions and is still used as a spiritual purification rite. Christianity, Judaism, Islam, Buddhism, Hinduism, and many tribal, anamistic religions have encouraged fasting as penance, preparation for ceremony, purification, mourning, sacrifice, divine union, and to enhance mental and spiritual powers. The Bible is filled with stories of people fasting for purification and communion with God. The Essenes, authors of the Dead Sea Scrolls, also advocated fasting as one of their primary methods of healing and spiritual revelation, as described in *The Essene Gospel of Peace* (translated by Edmond Bordeaux Szekely from the third-century Aramaic manuscript).

Philosophers, scientists, and physicians across time have fasted as a means to promote life and health after sickness. Socrates, Plato, Aristotle, Galen, Paracelsus, and Hippocrates all used fasting therapy. Many of today's spiritual teachers also recommend fasting as a useful tool. In a lecture entitled "Healing by God's Unlimited Power" (1947), Paramahansa Yogananda suggested that fasting increased our natural resistance to disease, stating that "Fasting is a natural method of healing. When animals or savages are sick, they fast. Most diseases can be cured by judicious fasting. Unless one has a weak heart, regular short fasts have been recommended by the yogis as an excellent health measure."

Through the centuries, physicians and healers have treated a variety of maladies with fasting, acknowledging that *ignorance of how to live in accordance with nature may be our greatest disease.* Our inherent knowledge of how to live according to the natural laws and spiritual truths leads to the sacred wisdom of life and subsequent good health. Knowing when and how long to fast is part of this knowledge. Through fasting, we can turn our energies inward, where we can use them for healing, clarity, and change.

Physicians with a spiritual orientation tend to be more inclined than others to employ fasting, both personally and in their practices. Many of my own life transitions were stimulated and supported through fasting; when I felt blocked or needed creative energy in my writing, fasting has been very useful. In *Spiritual Nutrition and the Rainbow Diet*, physician and spiritual teacher Gabriel Cousens, M.D., includes an excellent chapter on fasting in which he describes his theories and his own 40-day regime. According to Dr. Cousens,

> *. . . fasting in a larger context, means to abstain from that which is toxic to mind, body, and soul. A way to understand this is that fasting is the elimination of physical, emotional, and mental toxins from our organism, rather than simply cutting down on or stopping food intake. Fasting for spiritual purposes usually involves some degree of removal of oneself from worldly responsibilities. It can mean complete silence and social isolation during the fast which can be a great revival to those of us who have been putting our energy outward.*

From a medical point of view, I believe that fasting is not utilized often enough. We take vacations from work to relax, recharge, and gain new perspectives on our life—why not take occasional breaks from food? (Or, for that matter, from excessive activity or television?) To break the habit of eating three meals a day is a challenge for most of us. When we stop and let our stomach remain empty, our body goes into an elimination cycle, and most people will experience some withdrawal symptoms, especially when toxicity exists. Symptoms include headaches, irritability, or fatigue. As with all allergy-addictions, eating again assuages these symptoms.

Fasting is a useful therapy for so many conditions and people. Those who tend to develop congestive symptoms do well with fasting; congestive acidic conditions include colds, flus, bronchitis, mucus congestion, and constipation. If not addressed, such conditions can lead to headaches, chronic intestinal problems, skin conditions, and more severe ailments. Most of us living in Western, industrialized nations suffer from both overnutrition and undernutrition. We take in excessive amounts of potentially toxic nutrients, such as fats and chemicals, and inadequate amounts of many essential vitamins and minerals. The resulting congestive diseases are characterized by excess mucus and sluggish elimination; deficiency problems result from either poor nourishment or ineffective digestion/assimilation. Juice fasting supplies nutrients while still allowing for the elimination of toxins.

Juice fasting can be used both to detoxify from drugs and when embarking on a new lifestyle transition provided there are no contraindications (discussed later in this chapter). Fasting is versatile and generally safe; however, when used to treat medical conditions, proper supervision should be employed. Many physicians, chiropractors, acupuncturists, and nutritionists feel comfortable overseeing people during fasting, and I encourage you to seek them out if your condition warrants supervision.

Do You Experience Any Of These Conditions For Which Fasting May Be Beneficial?		
colds	environmental allergies	diabetes
flus	asthma	fever
bronchitis	insomnia	fatigue
headaches	skin conditions	back pains
constipation	atherosclerosis	mental illness
indigestion	coronary artery disease	obesity
diarrhea	angina pectoris	cancer
food allergies	hypertension	epilepsy

• The use of fasting as a treatment for **fevers** is controversial. It shouldn't be. Consuming liquids generates less heat, and this helps cool the body. With fever, we need more liquids than usual.

• Some cases of **fatigue** respond well to fasting, particularly when the fatigue results from congested organs and stalled energy. With fatigue that results from chronic infection, nutritional deficiency, or serious disease, added nourishment is probably called for as opposed to fasting.

• **Back pain** caused by muscular tightness and stress (rather than from bone disease or osteoporosis) are usually alleviated with a lighter diet or juice fasting. Much tightness and soreness along the back results from colon or other organ congestion; in my experience, poor bowel function and constipation are commonly associated with back pain.

• Patients with **mental illness** ranging from anxiety to schizophrenia may be helped by fasting. Although this may sound sensational, fasting's purpose here, however, is not to cure these problems, but rather to help understand the relationship of foods, chemicals, and drugs with mental functioning. Additional allergies and environmental reactions are not at all uncommon in people with mental illness. True, the release of toxins or lack of nourishment during fasting may worsen psychiatric problems; if, however, the patient is strong and congested, fasting may be helpful. The supervision of a healthcare provider is important for patients with mental illness.

- People often attempt to remedy **obesity** by fasting, although it is not the best use of this healing technique. Fasting is actually too temporary an approach for overweight dieters and may even generate feasting reactions in people coming off the fast. A better solution would be a more gradual change of diet with a longer-term weight-reduction plan—something that will replace old dietary habits and food choices with new ones. However, a short 5- to 10-day fast can motivate people to make the necessary dietary changes and renewed commitments to proper eating.

  Some very obese patients who have needed to shed weights of a hundred pounds or more have been on month-long water fasts supervised in hospitals. Other patients have had their jaws wired shut allowing them to only ingest fluids through straws. Newer fasting programs substitute a variety of protein-rich powders for meals. These are also usually medically supervised, and are for people who are at least 30–50 pounds overweight. These high-protein, low-calorie diets (using prepackaged powders such as Optifast or Medifast) allow patients to burn more fat. Although these programs are not nearly as healthful as vital juice fasts, they are more nutritionally supportive over a longer period of time and can be used on a outpatient basis fairly safely if people are monitored regularly. They provide all the needed vitamins, minerals, and amino acids to sustain life while helping many people lower their weight, blood fats, blood pressure, and blood sugars. However, as with any weight-loss program, success depends upon participant motivation to change personal diets and habits permanently, as fluctuating weights may actually be more harmful than just remaining overweight. Many obese people are also deficient in nutrients because they eat a highly refined, fatty, sweet diet. They are often fatigued and need to be nourished first before they will do well on any fast. A well-balanced, low-calorie (yet high-nutrient) diet with lots of exercise is still the best way to reduce and maintain a good weight and figure.

- Fasting to treat **cancer** is a controversial topic but is used by many alternative clinics outside the United States. Because of cancer's extremely debilitating effects, this may not be wise. Juice fasting may be helpful in early stages of cancer, and is definitely a preventative measure as it reduces toxicity. Anyone with cancer needs adequate nourishment; adding fresh juices to an already wholesome diet can promote mild detoxification and enhance overall vitality.

The Process and Benefits of Fasting

Although the results of fasting will vary depending upon the individual condition of the faster, there are a number of metabolic changes and experiences that are common to all. First, fasting is a catalyst for change and an essential part of transformational medicine. It promotes relaxation and energization of the body, mind, and emotions, and supports a greater spiritual awareness. Many fasters let go of past experiences and develop a positive attitude toward the present. Having plenty of energy to get things done and cleaning up our personal and community environment is also a common response to the cleansing process. Fasting definitely improves motivation and stimulates creative energy; it also enhances health, beauty, and vitality by letting many of the body systems rest.

Fasting is a multidimensional experience, affecting people physically, mentally, emotionally, and spiritually. Breaking down stored or circulating chemicals is its basic process; the blood and lymph also have the opportunity to be cleaned of toxins as their eliminative functions are alleviated. Each cell has the opportunity to catch up on its work; with fewer new demands, cells can repair themselves and eliminate wastes. Most fasters experience a new vibrancy of their skin and clarity of mind and body. Most importantly, our liver can spend more time detoxifying our body and creating new essential substances. Two to three quarts of water and juices daily (or even more in some people) are optimal during fasting to cleanse and support our body.

Metabolically, fasting initially reduces caloric intake to the point where the liver converts stored glycogen to glucose and energy. Body fat and fatty acids can be used for energy (ATP); however, the brain and central nervous system need direct glucose. With fasting, some protein breakdown occurs (less if calories are provided by juices). When glycogen stores are low, our body can convert protein to amino acids and to energy—specifically the amino acids alanine and serine can be used to produce glucose. Fatty acids can also be a source of energy during fasting, as they convert to ketones (acetone bodies) which can be used by the body to prevent protein loss. With juice fasting, there is less ketosis (disrupted carbohydrate metabolism) and the simple carbohydrates provided by the juices are easily used for energy and cellular function. High-protein (fasting) diets and other weight-loss programs may burn more fat and generate more ketosis, but they also add more toxins and may create other health concerns.

Fasting increases the process of elimination and the release of toxins from the colon, kidneys, bladder, lungs, sinuses, and skin. This process can generate discharges such as mucus which are helpful in clearing biochemical suffocation. Fasting helps us decrease this suffocation by allowing the cells to eliminate waste products, increase oxygenation, and improve cellular nutrition.

SOME BENEFITS OF FASTING	
Purification	Drug detoxification
Rejuvenation	Better resistance to disease
More energy	Spiritual awareness
Rest for digestive organs	More restful sleep
Greater abdominal peace	More relaxation
Clearer skin	Greater motivation and optimism
Sense of personal beauty	New inspiration and creativity
Anti-aging effects	More clarity, mental and emotional
Improved senses—vision, hearing, taste	Improved communications
Self-confidence	Better organization
Reduction of allergies	Clean personal space
Weight loss	Commitment to habit changes
Clothes fit more comfortably	Diet changes, long term

As for fasting symptoms, headache is not at all uncommon during the first day or two. Hunger is usually present for two or three days and then departs, leaving many people with a surprising feeling of deep "abdominal peace." When hungry, it is good to ask ourselves, "What are we hungry for?" Fasting is an excellent time to work on the psychological aspects of consumption. Fatigue or irritability may arise at times, as may dizziness or lightheadedness. Sensitivity is usually increased, and common sounds like the telephone, television, music, or the hum of a refrigerator or air-conditioner may be more irritating. Our sense of smell is also exaggerated. Most people's tongues will develop a thick white or yellow fur coating, which can be scraped or brushed off. Bad breath and displeasing tastes in the mouth, or foul-smelling urine or stools, may occur. Skin odor or skin eruptions such as small spots or painful boils may also appear, depending on the level of toxicity. Digestive upset, mucus-containing stools, flatulence, or even nausea and vomiting may also occur. Some people experience insomnia or bad dreams as their body releases poisons during the night. Believe me, the ultimate benefits are well worth the transient discomforts.

The mind may put up resistance, sending messages of doubt or fear that fasting is not right. This can be exaggerated by listening to other people's fears about your fasting. (If you are looking for excuses not to fast, they are everywhere.) Most symptoms will occur early on (if at all) and will pass. Generally, energy levels are good, although energy may go down every two or three days as the body excretes more wastes. It is at these times that resistance and fears (as well as new symptoms) may arise; if symptoms occur, it is wise to drink more fluids. However, most people will feel cleaner, better, and more alive most of the time.

Old symptoms or patterns from the past may arise during fasts—again usually transiently—or new symptoms of detoxification may appear. This "crisis" or periodic cleansing is not predictable and often raises doubts and questions—is this a new problem or part of the healing process? Generally, time and the healing process will sort things out. We should use Hering's Law of Cure to guide us in making these judgment calls. It states that healing happens from the inside out, the top down, from more important organs to less important ones, and from the most recent to the oldest symptoms. Most healing crises pass within a day or two, although some cleansers experience several days of "cold" symptoms or sinus congestion. If any symptom lasts longer than two or three days, it should be considered a side effect or new problem and should be addressed accordingly. If a problem worsens or causes concern (fainting, heart arrythmias, or bleeding) the fast should be stopped and a doctor consulted.

Medical supervision is important for anyone in poor health or without fasting experience. If the fast is extended for more than three or four days, regular monitoring, including physical examinations and blood work, should be done weekly (particularly if there is any cause for concern). Fasting may reduce blood protein levels and will definitely lower blood fats. Uric acid levels may rise due to protein breakdown, while levels of some minerals such as potassium, sodium, calcium, or magnesium may drop. Iron levels are usually lower, and the red blood cell count may also drop slightly during this time. Lowered mineral levels can result in fatigue or muscle cramps; if these should occur, additional minerals, (particularly calcium, magnesium, and potassium) should be taken, ideally in a powered form for easy assimilation.

Nutritionally, fasting helps us appreciate the more subtle aspects of our diet, as less food and simple flavors will become more satisfying (even food aromas can be fulfilling). Mentally, fasting improves clarity and attentiveness; emotionally, it may make us more sensitive and aware of our feelings. I have seen individuals gain the clarity to make important decisions during this therapy. Fasting definitely supports the transformational, evolutionary process. Juice fasting offers a lesson in self-restraint and control of passions. This new and empowering sense of self-discipline can be highly motivating. Fasters who were once spectators suddenly become doers.

Hazards of Fasting

If fasting is overused, it may create depletion and weakness in the body, lowering resistance and increasing susceptibility to disease. While fasting does allow the organs, tissues, and cells to rest and handle excesses, the body needs the nourishment provided by food to function after it has used up its stores.

Malnourished people should definitely not fast, nor should some overweight people who are undernourished. Others who should not fast include people with fatigue resulting from nutrient deficiency, those with chronic degenerative disease of the muscles or bones, or those who are underweight. Diseases associated with clogged or toxic organs respond better to fasting. Sluggish individuals who retain water or whose weight is concentrated in their hips and legs often do worse. Those with low daytime energy and more vitality at night (more yin or alkaline types) may not enjoy fasting either.

I do not recommend fasting for pregnant or lactating women, or for people who have weak hearts, or weakened immunity. (I have, however, seen women use short juice cleanses during their menstrual cycle to help ease pain and other symptoms.) Before or after surgery is not a good time to fast, as the body needs its nourishment to handle the stress and healing demands of the operation. Although some nutritional therapies for cancer include medically-supervised fasting, I do not recommend it for cancer patients, particularly those with advanced problems. Ulcer disease is not something for which I usually suggest fasting, either, although fasting may be beneficial for other conditions present in a patient whose ulcer is under control.

Some clinics and fasting practitioners do believe in fasting for ulcers. In the first test case of the Master Cleanser (p. 119), Stanley Burroughs claims to have cured a patient with an intractable ulcer. The two main ingredients of the Master Cleanser, citrus and cayenne pepper, are substances which all the physicians had suggested this patient avoid; Dr. Burroughs deduced they might be the only things left to heal the ulcer, and perhaps he is right. The fasting process itself is helpful for ulcers as it reduces stomach acid and aids in tissue healing. Cayenne pepper, although hot, heals mucous membranes and is commonly recommended for ulcers in herbal medicines. So, even though peptic ulcers are on the contraindication list, some people may be helped by fasting, especially with cabbage/vegetable juices.

CONTRAINDICATIONS FOR FASTING

Underweight	Low blood pressure	Pre- and postsurgery
Fatigue	Cardiac arrythmias	Cancer
Low immunity	Cold weather	Peptic ulcers
Weak heart	Pregnancy	Nutritional deficiencies
	Nursing	

As with any therapy, fasting has some potential hazards. Clearly, excessive weight loss and nutritional deficiencies may occur—a response more marked with longer water fasts and less likely with juices as they provide some calories and nutrients. Weakness may occur, or muscle cramps may result from mineral deficits. Sodium, potassium, calcium, magnesium, and phosphorus losses occur initially but diminish after a week. Blood pressure drops, and this can lead to dizziness (especially when changing position from lying to sitting or from sitting to standing). Uric acid levels may rise without adequate fluid intake, although this is rare.

Some research reports hormone level changes while fasting. Initially, the level of thyroid hormone falls, but it rises again in association with protein-sparing ketosis. Female hormone levels fall, possibly as a result of protein malnutrition, and this can lead to a lessening or loss of menstrual flow. Cessation of periods in women is also seen in longtime vegetarians, particularly those who exercise extensively, arising I believe from nutrient depletion. This will usually rebalance with proper diet and nourishment.

Cardiac problems such as arrhythmias can occur with prolonged fasting, especially when there are preexisting problems. Extra beats, both ventricular and atrial, have been seen, and there have even been deaths from serious ventricular arrhythmias (the latter of which occur most often during long water fasts). Similar problems have turned up in people using any nutrient-deficient protein powders, without supervision, as a weight loss tool. All of these risks are minimized with juice fasts of no more than two weeks duration, or when basic minerals (potassium, calcium, and magnesium) are supplemented during water fasts. Having our progress monitored through physical exams, blood tests, and even electrocardiograms is another way to protect ourselves from fasting's potential hazards.

Another "side effect" of fasting is the way it affects and changes our personal lives. Often we resist inner guidance, feelings, and desires to do something new or get out of a bad situation, but fasting brings them to the fore. Divorce, job changes, and residential moves are all more likely after fasts, as they stimulate self-realization, enhance our potential, and help us focus on the future. During fasting, many people have new sensitivity and renewed awareness of their job, mate, and home. I usually warn fasters before they begin of the great potential for change, especially when I sense that they lack commitment or belief in what they are doing. Even though these insights and changes may be traumatic initially, I believe they are ultimately positive and help us follow our true nature.

How to Fast

The general plan for fasting is progressive, usually a moderate approach for new fasters and unhealthy subjects and leading to a stricter program for the more experienced. It is important to build slowly and take time to transition. Although many people do fine even when making extreme changes, such abruptness clearly maximizes the risks of fasting.

A sensible daily plan mixes fasting with eating. Each day can include a 12–14 hour period of fasting from early evening through the night, as indeed breakfast was given that name to denote the time where we *break the fast* of the night. Many people eat very lightly or not at all in the early morning in order to extend their daily fast; this is more important if dinner or snacking extends into the later evening. However, if dinner is at an early time, a good breakfast can be consumed after water intake and some exercise.

In preparation for our first day of fasting, we may want to take some time (a few days to a week) to eliminate unhealthy foods or habits from our diet. Abstaining from alcohol, nicotine, caffeine, and sugar is very helpful before fasting. Red meats and other animal foods, including milk products and eggs, could be avoided for a day or two before fasting, thus easing the transition. Intake of most nutritional supplements should be also be curtailed as these are usually not recommended during a fast. Many people prepare for their fasts by consuming only fruit and vegetable foods for three or four days. These slowly detoxify the body so that the actual fast will be less intense.

The first one-day fast gives us a chance to see what a short fast can be like. Most of us find that it is not so very difficult and does not cause major distress. Food is abstained from for 36 hours, from 8 PM one night until 8 AM two days later. Most people will feel a little hungry and may experience a few mild symptoms such as a headache or irritability by the end of the fasting day, usually around dinnertime. The first two days are generally challenging for everyone; feeling great usually begins around day three. So take a walk, take a nap, cut your nails, read a book, pray, and bathe instead of eating.

One of the ironies of fasting is that it can be the most difficult for those who need it the most; in these cases, people must start with the subtle diet changes discussed above. One transition protocol is the one-meal-a-day plan. The meal is usually eaten around 3 PM; water, juices, teas, and some fresh fruit or vegetable snacks can be eaten at other times. It is important that the wholesome meal be neither excessive nor rich. I suggest a protein and vegetable meal, such as fish and salad or steamed vegetables, or a starch and vegetable meal, such as brown rice and mixed steamed greens, carrots, celery, and zucchini. People on this plan start to detoxify slowly, lose some weight, and after a few days feel pretty sound. The chance of any strong symptoms developing during this transition time or during a subsequent fast is greatly minimized.

The next goal for those who have done a one-meal-a-day program is a one-day fast. The fasting then progresses to two- and three-day fasts with one or two days between them when light foods and more raw fruits and vegetables are consumed. This allows us to build up to longer lasting five- to ten-day fasts. When the transition is made this slowly, even a water fast can be less intense (although I usually recommend juice fasts).

To avoid being excessively impatient, we need to make and adhere to a plan. It is important to continually observe and listen to our body and maybe keep notes in a journal. Get to know yourself and your nature. Once we have fasted successfully, we can continue to do one-day fasts weekly or a three-day fast every month if we need them. This experience helps us to reconnect with ourselves and to work toward a goal of optimum health. Meditation, exercise, fresh air and sunshine, massages, and baths are all essential and nourishing during this and any cleansing period.

Timing of Fasts

The two key times for natural cleansing are the times of transition into Spring and Autumn. In Chinese medicine, this transition time between the seasons is about ten days before and after each equinox or solstice. For spring, this period runs from about March 10 through April 1; for autumn, it is from about September 11 through October 2. In cooler climates, where spring weather begins later and autumn weather earlier, the fasting could be scheduled appropriately as it is easier to do when it is warm as the body tends to cool down during fasting.

For a spring fast, I usually suggest lemon and/or greens as the focus of the cleansing. Diluted lemon water, lemon and honey, or, my favorite, the Master Cleanser, can be used.

SPRING MASTER CLEANSER

2 Tablespoons fresh lemon or lime juice
1 Tablespoon pure maple syrup (up to 2 tablespoons if you want to drop less weight)
1/10 teaspoon cayenne pepper
8 ounces spring water

Mix and drink 8–12 glasses throughout the day. Eat or drink nothing else except water, laxative herb tea, and peppermint or chamomile tea. Keep the Cleanser in a glass container (not plastic) or make it fresh each time. Rinse your mouth with water after each glass to prevent the lemon juice from hurting the enamel of your teeth.

Fresh fruit or vegetable juices diluted with equal amounts of water will also stimulate cleansing. Some good vegetable choices are carrots, celery, beets, and greens. Soup broths can also be used. Juices with blue-green algae, spirulina, or chlorella provide more energy, as they contain quality protein (amino acids) and are easily assimilated.

In autumn, a fast of at least 3 to 5 days can be done, using either water or a variety of juices. Juices could include the Master Cleanser, apple and/or grape juice (usually mixed with a little lemon and water to reduce sweetness), vegetable juices, and warm broths.

AUTUMN REJUVENATION RATION*

3 cups spring water
1 Tablespoon ginger root, chopped
1–2 Tablespoons miso paste (do not boil)
1–2 stalks green onion, chopped

cilantro, to taste, chopped
1–2 pinches cayenne pepper
2 teaspoons olive oil
juice of 1/2 lemon

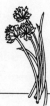

Boil water. Add ginger root. Simmer 10 minutes. Stir in miso paste to taste. Turn off burner. Then add green onion, some cilantro, cayenne, olive oil, and lemon juice. Remove and cover to steep for 10 minutes. May vary ingredient portions to satisfy flavors. Enjoy

* From Bethany ArgIsle

How do we know how long to fast?

We can either follow a specific time schedule, or listen closely to our own individual cycles and needs. Paying attention to our energy level, degree of congestion, and observing of our tongue and its coating will offer helpful cleansing guidelines. As we gain some fasting experience, we will become more attuned to specific times when we need to strengthen or lighten our diet and when we need to cleanse. If we are under stress, have been overindulging, or develop some congestive symptoms, we need to lighten our diet and possibly cleanse. The odor of our urine, breath, and sweat are telltale signs of cleansing in action.

Breaking a Fast

Ending or stopping a fast and beginning to eat again also takes some monitoring. Things to watch include energy level, weight, detox symptoms, tongue coating, and degree of hunger. If our energy falls for more than a day or if our weight gets too low, we should come off the fast. If symptoms are particularly intense or sudden, it is possible that we need food. Generally, the tongue is a good indicator of our state of toxicity or clarity. With fasting, the tongue usually becomes coated with a white, yellow, or gray film. This signals the body's cleansing process, and it will usually clear when the detox cycle is complete. However, tongue observation is not a foolproof indicator. Some people's tongues may coat very little, while others will remain coated even after cleansing. If in doubt, it is better to make the transition back to food and then cleanse again later. Hunger is another sign of readiness to move back into eating, as it is often minimal during cleansing times. Occasionally, people are very hungry throughout a fast, but most lose interest in food from day three to seven and then experience real, deep-seated hunger once again. This is a sign to eat carefully.

Breaking a fast must be well planned and executed slowly and carefully to prevent the creation of symptoms and sickness. It is suggested that we take half of our total cleansing time to move back into our regular diet, which is hopefully now better planned and more healthful. Our digestion has been at rest, so we need to chew our foods very well. If we have fasted on water alone, we need to prepare our digestive tract with diluted juices, perhaps beginning with a few teaspoons of fresh orange juice in a glass of water and progressing to stronger mixtures throughout the day. Diluted fresh grape or orange juice will stimulate the digestion. Arnold Ehret, a European fasting expert and proponent of the "mucusless" diet, suggests that fruits and fruit juices should not be used right after a meat eater's first fast because they may coagulate intestinal mucus and cause problems. A meat eater's colon bacteria are probably different from a vegetarian's. Consequently, fruit sugars like those in the juices may not be tolerated; instead, the active gram-positive anaerobic bacteria in the meat eater will produce more toxins. Extra acidophilus supplements continued on a regular basis help shift colon ecology in meat eaters, and can even be used during cleanses.

With juice fasting, it is easier to transition back to food. A raw or cooked low-starch vegetable, such as spinach or other greens, is quite appropriate. A little sauerkraut also helps to stimulate the digestive function. A laxative-type meal including grapes, cherries, or soaked or stewed prunes can also be used to initiate eating, as they keep the bowels moving. Some experts say that the bowels should move within an hour or two after the first meal and, if not, an enema should be used. Some people do a saltwater flush before their first day of food by drinking a quart of water containing 2 teaspoons of dissolved sea salt. Be careful. Our individual transit times vary in response to laxatives and saltwater.

However you make the transition, go slowly, chew well, and do not overeat or mix too many foods at any meal. Start with simple vegetable meals, salads. Fruit should be eaten alone. Soaked prunes or figs are helpful. Well-cooked, watery brown rice or millet is handled well by most people by the second day. From there, progress slowly through grains and vegetables. Some nuts, seeds, or legumes can be added, and then richer protein foods, if these are desired. Returning to food is a crucial time for learning individual responses or reactions. Self-observation gives us an opportunity to see destructive dietary habits and discover specific food intolerances. You may wish to keep notes at this time. If you respond poorly to a food, avoid it for a week or so, and then eat it alone to see how it feels. This is when food allergies may be revealed.

Juice Specifics

Some juices work better for certain people or conditions. In general, diluted fresh juices of raw organic fruits and vegetables are best. Canned and frozen juices should be avoided. Some bottled juice may be used, but fresh squeezed or extracted is best, as long as it is used soon after processing. Lemon juice, wheat grass, or a little ginger or garlic juice can be added to drinks for vitality and to stimulate cleansing.

Water and other liquids increase waste elimination. Lemon tends to loosen and draw out mucus and is especially useful for liver cleansing. Diluted lemon juice with or without a little honey or the Master Cleanser lemonade loosens mucus quickly, so if this is used we need to cleanse the bowels regularly to prevent getting sick. Most vegetable juices are milder than lemon juice.

Each juice has a certain nutritional composition and probable physiological actions (although these have not been studied extensively). Fresh juices are like natural vitamin pills with a very high assimilation rate which do not require the work of digestion.

The juices of apples, grapes, oranges, and carrots are good cleansing juices but might be minimized for weight loss as they are high in calories. Juices more helpful for weight loss include grapefruit, lemon, cucumber, and greens such as lettuce, spinach, or parsley. Also, a variety of juices can be used in a fast, prepared fresh daily. Keep recipes of your favorite new combinations.

FRUIT JUICES	VEGETABLE JUICES
Lemon—liver, gallbladder, allergies, asthma, cardiovascular disease (CVD), colds	**Greens**—CVD, skin, eczema, digestive problems, obesity, breath
Citrus—CVD, obesity, hemorrhoids, varicose veins	**Spinach**—anemia, eczema
Apple—liver, intestines	**Parsley**—kidneys, edema, arthritis
Pear—gallbladder	**Beet greens**—gallbladder, liver, osteoporosis
Grape—colon, anemia	**Watercress**—anemia, colds
Papaya—stomach, indigestion, hemorrhoids, colitis	**Wheat grass**—anemia, liver, intestines, breath
Pineapple—allergies, arthritis, inflammation, edema, hemorrhoids	**Cabbage**—colitis, ulcers
Watermelon—kidneys, edema	**Comfrey**—intestines, hypertension, osteoporosis
Black cherry—colon, menstrual problems, gout	**Carrots**—eyes, arthritis, osteoporosis
	Beets—blood, liver, menstrual problems, arthritis
	Celery—kidneys, diabetes, osteoporosis
	Cucumber—edema, diabetes
	Jerusalem artichokes—diabetes
	Garlic—allergies, colds, hypertension, CVD, high fats, diabetes
	Radish—liver, high fats, obesity
	Potatoes—intestines, ulcers

To prepare juices, we want to start with the freshest and most chemical-free fruits and vegetables possible. They should be cleaned or soaked and stored properly. If not organic, they should be peeled, especially if they are waxed. With root vegetables such as carrots or beets, the above-ground ends should be trimmed. Some people drop their vegetables into a pot of boiling water for a minute or so to clean them before juicing. If there is a question of toxicity, sprays, or parasites, a chlorine bleach bath can be used.

Soaking fresh foods in small amounts of Clorox bleach (sodium hypoclorite) can help break down pesticide chemicals and disinfect the food from parasites or other potentially harmful microorganisms. In a sink, add about one tablespoon of Clorox bleach per gallon of water and soak your fruits and vegetables for about 15-30 minutes. Rinse and follow with two soaks of water only for 30 minutes each before drying and storing.

The right juicer is important. The rotary-blade juicers (Champion brand) are very good at squeezing the juice with minimum molecular irritation and are medium in price range. The centrifuge juicers are also fine, but they waste juice left in pulp. The best juicers are the compressors (Norwalk brand) which are more expensive. Blenders are not really juicers; what they produce is more like liquid salad. These drinks can also be used for a fast since they are high in fiber and nutrients. I once did a energizing week-long fast with two blender drinks a day—fruits in the morning and vegetables in the late afternoon—with teas and water in between.

Other Aspects of Healthy Fasting

- **Fresh air**—plenty is needed to support cleansing and oxygenation of the cells and tissues.
- **Sunshine**—also needed to revitalize our body; avoid excessive exposure.
- **Water**—bathing is very important to cleanse the skin at least twice daily.
- **Steams** and **saunas** are also good for providing warmth and supporting detoxification.
- **Skin brushing**—with a dry, soft brush prior to bathing is a good year-round practice as well. This will help clear toxins from the skin.
- **Exercise**—very important to support the cleansing process. It helps to relax the body, clears wastes, and prevents toxicity symptoms. Walking, bicycling, swimming, or other exercise can be done during a fast, although sports which entail risk, danger, or physical contact should be avoided.

- **No drugs**—none should be used during fasts except mandatory prescription drugs. Avoidance of alcohol, nicotine, and caffeine is imperative.

- **Vitamin supplements**—these are not used during fasting and thus no program of nutrients will follow at the end of this chapter. Supplemental fiber, such as psyllium husks, can help detox the colon. Special chlorophyll foods such as green barley, chlorella, spirulina, or blue-green algae may enhance vitality and purification. Occasionally, some mineral support (especially potassium, calcium, magnesium, with vitamin C) in powdered or liquid forms helps prevent cramps or adds support during an extended fast. Some people even use amino-acid or other vitamin powders. These supplemental nutrients are really best used when consumed with foods.

- **Colon cleansing**—an essential part of healthy fasting. Some form of bowel stimulation is recommended. Colonic irrigations with water performed by a trained therapist with modern equipment are the most thorough. These can be done at the beginning, midpoint, and end of the fast. It is suggested that enemas be used at least every other day, especially if they are the primary cleansing method. Fasting clinics often suggest that enemas be used daily or several times a day. With these, water alone is used to flush the colon of toxins. It may be helpful for an enema or laxative preparation to be used the day before the fast begins to lessen initial toxicity. Herbal laxatives are commonly taken orally during fasting, and many formulas are available either as capsules or for making tea. These include cascara sagrada, senna leaves, licorice root, buckthorn, rhubarb root, aloe vera, and prepared formulas. The salt-water flush (drinking a quart of warm water with two teaspoons of sea salt dissolved in it) can be used first thing in the morning on alternate days throughout the fast to flush the entire intestinal tract, although it does not work well for everyone. It is not recommended for salt-sensitive or water-retaining people, or for hypertensives.

- **Work and be creative**—and make plans for your life. Staying busy helps break our ties to food. Most fasters experience greater work energy and more creativity and, naturally, find lots to do.

- **Cleanup**—both our body and our environment: our room, desk, office, closet, and home. If we want to prepare for the new, we need to clear out the old.

- **Joining others** in fasting can generate strong bonds and provide an additional spiritual lift. It creates new supportive relationships and adds levels to existing ones. Most people feel better as their fast progresses—more vital, lighter, less blocked, more flexible, clearer, and more spiritually attuned. For many, it is nice to have someone with whom to share this. Call our clinic or another that offers this service.

- **Avoid the negative influence of others** who may not understand or support us. Remember to listen to your inner guidance and to be aware of any problems. Being in contact with other fasters or sympathetic people who understand fasting's benefits will provide us with the positive, grounded support we need.
- The economy of fasting allows us to **save time, money, and future health care costs.** Many of us will be inspired to share more of ourselves when we are freed from food.
- **Meditation and relaxation** are other important aspects of fasting which help clear stresses and bring us into contact with ourselves.
- **Spiritual practice and prayer** will affirm our positive attitude and support our meditation and relaxation, providing us with inner fuel to live with purpose and passion.

Conclusion

When we overdo it with food or other substances, we need to return to the cycle of a daily night fast of 12–14 hours and eating one main meal and two lighter ones. For low-weight, high-metabolism people, two larger- or three moderately-sized meals are probably needed. If we eat a heavier evening meal, we may need only a light breakfast, and vice versa. Through awareness and experience, we can find our individual nutritional needs and fulfill them with ease.

Fasting can easily become both a way of life and an effective dietary practice. Over a period of time we can go from symptom cleansing to preventive fasting. We should support ourselves regularly with a balanced, wholesome diet, and fast at specific times to treat symptoms and/or to enhance our vitality and spiritual practice. If we could devote one day per week to purification and a cleansing diet, the path of health would be smooth indeed.

Choosing healthy foods, chewing well, and maintaining good colon function all minimize our need for fasting. However, if we do get out of balance, we can employ one of the oldest treatments known to humans, the instinctive therapy for many illnesses, nature's doctor, therapist, and tool for preventing disease—FASTING!

(Books that are out of print might be obtainable through your local library.)

Aero, Rita and Stephanie Rick. *Vitamin Power: A User's Guide to Nutritional Supplements and Botanical Substances That Can Change Your Life.* New York: Harmony Books, 1987. (Out of print.)

Airola, Paavo. *How to Get Well.* Phoenix, AZ: Health Plus, 1981. (Out of print.)

Bland, Dr. Jeffrey. *The 20-Day Rejuvenation Diet Program.* New Canaan, CT: Keats Publishing, Inc., 1996.

Casdorph, H. Richard, M.D., and Morton Walker, M.D. *Toxic Metal Syndrome: How Metal Poisonings Can Affect Your Brain.* Garden City Park, NY: Avery Publishing Group, 1995.

Cousens, Gabriel, M.D. *Spiritual Nutritional and the Rainbow Diet.* San Rafael, CA: Cassandra Press, 1986.

Dadd, Debra Lynn. *Nontoxic Home and Office: Protecting Yourself and Your Family from Every-day Toxins and Health Hazards, rev. ed.* Los Angeles, CA: Jeremy P. Tarcher, 1992.

Dadd, Debra Lynn. *Nontoxic, Natural, and Earthwise: How to Protect Yourself from Harmful Products and Live in Harmony with the Earth.* Los Angeles, CA: Jeremy P. Tarcher, 1990.

Dufty, William. *Sugar Blues.* New York: Warners, 1966.

Ferguson, Tom, M.D. *Smoker's Book of Health: How to Keep Yourself Healthier and Reduce Your Smoking Risks.* New York: G. P. Putnam's Sons, 1987. (Out of print.)

Furman, Joel, M.D. *Fasting and Eating for Health.* New York: St. Martin's Press, 1995.

Gittleman, Ann Louise. *Guess What Came to Dinner: Parasites and Your Health.* Garden City Park, NY: Avery Publishing Group, 1993.

Pearson, Durk and Sandy Shaw. *Life Extension.* New York: Warner Books, 1987.

Reno, Liz and Joanna Devrais. *Allergy-Free Eating.* Berkeley, CA: Celestial Arts, 1995.

Saifer, Phyllis, M.D. *Detox.* Los Angeles, CA: Jeremy P. Tarcher, 1984. (Out of print.)

Silver, Helene. *Body Smart System: The Complete Guide to Cleansing and Rejuvenation, rev. ed.* Sonora, CA: Healthy Healing, 1995.

Sharp, Jim. *Basic Principles of Total Health: Harmonious Integration of Body, Mind, and Spirit.* Self-published. Call 510-287-5439 for info.

Shelton, Herbert. *Fasting Can Save Your Life.* Tampa, FL: American Natural Hygiene Society, 1978.

Szekely, Edmund Bordeaux. *The Essene Gospel of Peace.* Book 1. San Diego, CA: Academy Books, 1977.

Tompkins, Peter, and Christopher Bird. *Secrets of the Soil.* New York: Harper Collins, 1989.

Yogananda, Paramahansa. *Healing by God's Unlimited Power.* Los Angeles, CA: Self Realization Fellowship, 1975. (Out of print.)

Laboratories for Detoxification Testing and Assessment

Great Smokies Diagnostic Laboratory
63 Zillicoa St.
Asheville, NC 28801
800-522-4762

Diagnos-Techs, Inc.
6620 S. 192nd Pl., J-104
Kent, WA 98032
800-878-3787

Doctor's Data Laboratories, Inc.
301 W. 101 Roosevelt Road
W. Chicago, IL 60185
800-323-2784

Meridian Valley Clinical Laboratory
24030-132nd Avenue S.E.
Kent, WA 98042
800-234-6825

Immunosciences Lab, Inc.
8730 Wilshire Blvd., #305
Beverly Hills, CA 90211
800-950-4686

Metametrix Medical Laboratory
5000 Peachtree Industrial Blvd., Suite 110
Nocross, GA 30071
800-221-4640

ACCU-CHEM Laboratories
990 N. Bowser Rd., #800
Richardson, TX 75081
800-747-2878

Practitioners & Facilities

Healthcare for the 21st Century
Adrienne Buffaloe, MD, Director
964 Third Avenue
New York, NY 10155
212-355-2315, Fax 212-355-4496

Tree of Life Rejuvenation Center
Gabriel Cousens, MD.
P.O. Box 1080
Patagonia, AZ 85624
602-394-2060, Fax 602-394-2099

Optimum Health Institute of San Diego
6970 Central Avenue
Lemon Grove, CA 91945
619-464-3346

American Natural Hygiene Society
P.O. Box 30630
Tampa, FL 33630

Canadian Natural Hygiene Society
P.O. Box 235, Station T
Toronto, Ontario, Canada M6B 4A1

Susan Smith Jones
Health Unlimited and Celebrate Life!
P.O. Box 49396
Los Angeles, CA 90049

Azure Acres
Uwe Gunnersen, Director
2264 Green Hill Rd.
Sebastopol, Ca 95472
707-823-3385

St. Helena Health Center
at St. Helena Hospital
Deer Park, CA 94576
800-454-HOPE

Sierra Tucson & OnSite AfterCare
16500 N. Lago del Oro Parkway
Tucson, AZ 85739
800-842-4487

Center for Conservative Therapy
Alan Goldhamer, D.C., Director
4310 Lichau Rd.
Penngrove, CA 94951
707-792-2325, Fax 707-586-5544

Hotlines

Alcohol and Drug Helpline
800-354-7089

Center for Substance Abuse Treatment Hotline
800-662-4357

Children of Alcoholics Foundation
800-359-2623

Service of National Helplines
800-COCAINE
800-9-HEROIN
888-MARIJUANA
800-HELP-11
800-CRISIS-9
800-662-HELP

National Clearinghouse for Alcohol and Drug Information
(800-729-6686

National Cocaine Hotline
800-362-2463

National Council on Alcoholism and Drug Dependence
800-622-2255

National Acupuncture Detox Association (NADA) Information Center
3220 N St. NW #27
Washington, DC 20007

Also by Elson Haas:

Staying Healthy with Nutrition
The definitive resource for understanding the significant role of nutrition in our health.
1,200 pages

Staying Healthy with the Seasons
Dr. Haas's popular first book, now in its 20th printing, is a classic, integrating Eastern and Western health systems with practical guidelines for nutrition, herbology and exercise.
252 pages

A Diet for All Seasons
Dr. Haas gives us expert guidelines for changing our focus to fresh, home-cooked meals, attuned to the seasons, with menu plans and over 150 recipes.
224 pages

Available from your local bookstore, or direct from Celestial Arts, P.O. Box 7123, Berkeley, CA 94707. For VISA, MasterCard, and American Express orders call 800-841-BOOK.

You may contact Dr. Elson Haas:
Preventive Medical Center of Marin, Inc.
25 Mitchell Blvd., Suite 8
San Rafael, CA 94903
415-472-2343, Fax 415-472-7636
email: emhaas@sonic.net